MW01036853

AUTHOR

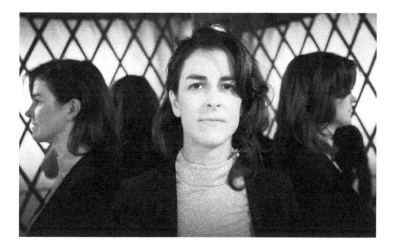

Georgeann Sack was awarded a PhD in Molecular, Cell, and Developmental Biology from the University of California, Los Angeles in 2011. She is Founder and Editor-in-Chief of *Awake & Alive Mind*, a publication on the science of consciousness. She lives in California with her husband and two children. This is her first book.

KEGELS ARE NOT GOING TO FIX THIS

The latest medical understanding
of pelvic floor disorders
and their impact on quality of life

GEORGEANN SACK

PUBLISHED BY AFFERENT, LLC
Davis, California, USA

Copyright © 2020 by Georgeann Sack

Thank you for buying an authorized edition of this book and complying with copyright laws. In doing so you are supporting the author. All rights reserved.

Contact georgeann@georgeannsack.com for permission to reproduce or distribute part of this publication.

Kegels Are Not Going to Fix This: The latest medical understanding of pelvic floor disorders and their impact on quality of life / Georgeann Sack

Library of Congress Control Number: 2020914240
ISBN 978-1-7350904-0-5 *(paperback)*
ISBN 978-1-7350904-1-2 *(ebook)*

Set in Adobe Caslon Pro with SPOT
Cover design by MiblArt
Author photo by Michael Poole
Additional photo and illustration credits on page 119

Dedicated to the mothers of the world.

To my children, Alice and Ivo. You are worth all of this and then some. Never doubt that you are loved.

CONTENTS

KEGELS ARE NOT GOING TO FIX THIS

"A RALLYING CRY"

L eaking urine and feces. Organs protruding from our bodies. Painful intercourse. Chronic discomfort. Pelvic floor disorders are medical problems resulting in diminished quality of life for one in three women around the world.

Though pelvic floor disorders are common, they should not be dismissed as "normal." There are a variety of medical treatment options, from surgery to nerve stimulation to physical therapy, that can alleviate or cure each disorder. There are also many ways to reduce your daily discomfort without ever seeing a doctor. I hope you will find this book a useful guide to care for your pelvic health and overall wellbeing.

I wrote this book for my sisters in suffering. I do not know your pain, but I know my own. To my horror, I discovered that my cervix and an unsightly bulge of vaginal tissue were protruding outside of my body following the birth of my first child. The lack of support or information from doctors added an extra level of stress and uncertainty that I could have done without.

For years, my doctors responded to my concerns as though they were temporary and not particularly significant. They were wrong. What I have aimed to do in this book is give you the information I wish I had from the beginning.

In addition to sharing lessons learned from my own experiences, I studied medical research literature to fill each chapter of this book with essential information every woman should know. Every woman benefits from becoming informed about her pelvic health and what symptoms to watch for.

The primary causes of pelvic floor disorders are giving birth and aging. I imagine a future where women are assessed for pelvic floor health during pre- and post-natal gynecological appointments and during each annual gynecological exam once they reach 50 years old. Those with symptoms would be referred to a urogynecologist for further assessment and treatment. Until then, this book is my attempt to fill the knowledge gap.

Chapter 1 provides an overview of the prevalence, risk factors, and anatomy of pelvic floor disorders. Chapter 2 takes an unflinching look at vaginal delivery as a physical trauma that can cause lasting damage. Chapter 3 unveils an underdiscussed reality of sexual dysfunction after vaginal delivery. Chapter 4 looks at the impact of pelvic floor disorders on quality of life. Chapter 5 investigates the efficacy of physical therapy for the treatment of pelvic floor disorders. Chapter 6 discusses the impact of additional pregnancies on pelvic floor disorders and explores the historical use of pessaries to provide relief for pelvic organ prolapse. Chapter 7 covers what is known about exercising with leaky or protruding pelvic organs. Chapter 8 is about the surgical treatment of pelvic floor disorders. Chapter 9 suggests new standard medical protocols that would provide comprehensive, holistic health care for women.

I decided to share my story because I felt alone in my problems. I wanted to give you at least one person's honest story so that you can feel less alone. My pelvic floor disorders ruined my ability to participate in some of life's basic pleasures — exercise and sex. They inflamed my vulva, such that I was in genital pain for at least half of each month. They gave me embarrassing problems with urinary incontinence and bowel movements that resulted in me being less engaged at work and in social situations.

When I first tried to share these problems with friends or doctors, their responses were casual, typically along the lines of, 'Yeah, vaginas change after giving birth. Have you tried Kegels?' They did not really get it, because these disorders hadn't happened to them. I was not sad that my vagina had changed, though that is deserving of mourning in itself. I was sad because I could not pee or poop normally. I leaked urine. Sex hurt. I had a bulge of tissue protruding from my body that created daily discomfort. I suspected that the damage sustained during childbirth went deeper than the vaginal tears that had been stitched up after delivery. Now I know that my connective tissues and muscles had torn off from their anchor points and were no longer performing their needed functions. I did not know this for certain until seven years after I gave birth, so I had only my intuition to rely on. I was broken, and Kegels were not going to fix it.

Writing this book was healing for me. My first draft was angry, full of blame, and probably not very interesting for anyone else to read. With each revision my personal story diminished as I became focused on getting quality information to others. I found myself trying to understand what it might be like for a 70 year old woman to notice that her cervix is starting to protrude from her body, or for a 25 year old woman to adjust to having fecal incontinence while caring for a newborn, or a 45 year old mother of 8 too busy to care for her leaking bladder or painful genitals even if there was adequate medical care nearby. I put in the work to help these imagined women, even though I did not have their exact problems.

Though women around the world have been coping with pelvic floor disorders since at least the earliest medical records and probably long before then, research related to pelvic floor disorders did not start in earnest until the 1980s. This change is largely due to the efforts of a small but persistent group of doctors who believed that the quality of care for women with pelvic floor disorders needed improvement.

In 1979, five doctors, a mix of gynecologists and urologists, founded what would become the American Urogynecologic Society, with annual meetings and their own research journal. Membership now exceeds 1,900, and there is also a thriving International Urogynecological Association. Leadership within the American Urogynecologic Society advocated for research funding and succeeded in convincing the U.S. National Institutes of Health *(NIH)* to fund research on pelvic floor disorders. The first dedicated NIH request for applications on pelvic floor disorders was in 1999. As a result, the number of published research papers on pelvic floor disorders has been steadily increasing over the last twenty years. There is finally evidence to drive needed changes in standard protocols for women's pelvic health.

Leadership within the Society also repeatedly made both informal and formal requests for subspecialty recognition and credentialed fellowships from the American Board of Obstetrics and Gynecology, a process that took 30 years.[1,2] As of 2011, Female Pelvic Medicine and Reconstructive Surgery is an accredited subspecialty with fellowships, exams, and certification. The first oral certifying exam was given in 2015.

The result of these changes is that there are more doctors with several years of additional training in the diagnosis and treatment of pelvic floor disorders. Their numbers will increase faster now that there is formalized training and credentialing.

It is interesting to look at this timeline alongside my own personal experience. I gave birth to my first child in 2012, when Female Pelvic Medicine and Reconstructive Surgery had just become an accredited subspecialty. The quality of my care was lacking. I gave birth to my second child in 2016. Within this short timeline, the quality of my care had improved. Perhaps this was a result of moving to a new town and the good luck of being placed with a gynecologist who happened to care about pelvic floor disorders. Or perhaps the formalized training had already started to have an impact, such that more gynecologists are knowledgeable about pelvic floor disorders and know to refer patients with incontinence or prolapse to urogynecologists.

Whatever the cause, I am grateful that these pioneers pushed for better care for women.

Let's not stop here. Now that the ball is rolling the real work can begin. In this book I offer ideas for changes I would like to see, but ultimately it is women's health doctors who need to agree upon a plan and push it into action.

As I was writing, I realized that I also want medical professionals to hear my story. If you are a gynecologist, urogynecologist, obstetrician, or pelvic floor physical therapist, this book is also for you. I think it is important for you to understand what these problems are like from the patient's perspective, which is something we rarely get a chance to share during our short appointments.

More than that, I want to encourage future doctors to enter these specialties. Women's health has a lot of room for improvement. If you want to be a leader or innovator, women's health provides a good opportunity to do so. If you want to dramatically change the quality of people's lives for the better, specializing in Female Pelvic Medicine would give you that chance daily. If you are interested in performing challenging surgeries that restore a woman's core bodily functions, consider reconstructive surgery for pelvic floor repair.

For a rallying cry from one of your own, consider this statement from M.D. and University of Michigan Professor John O.L. DeLancey.[3]

"Why should we care about this? For millennia, women have paid a lifelong price for their unique role in vaginal delivery, and we as obstetricians and gynecologists are responsible for their care. Given the remarkable scientific tools at our disposal, what is our generation doing to create a safer way for women to give birth?"

I consider this book a lighting of the torch, but I am not qualified to carry this torch alone. I am not a medical doctor. I am a scientist and a writer. My hope is that someone, or a great many someones, will read this book and be inspired to carry the torch.

One of my children is a girl. Someday she might want to have children of her own. I hope for her, and for all our girls, that we can give the next generation a better experience.

ACKNOWLEDGMENTS

I want to thank Dr. Andrew Walter for his feedback on an earlier draft of this book. Brooke Dulka for her excellent edits. Carolina Wonder Ehrlich for discussions about muscle systems, physical therapy, and integrating Kegels with yoga. Selene Fable, Katie Yurcich, Georgia Wade, Carolina Wonder Ehrlich, Esther Wright, and Caroline "Funshine" Meeks for reading an earlier draft and letting me know their thoughts.

Thank you to Doctors Don Ostergard, Jack Robertson, Andy Fantl, Henry Thiede, Linda Cardozo, Axel Ingelman-Sundberg, Ulf Ulmsten, Oscar Contreras Ortiz, John O.L. DeLancey, and so many others who recognized that health care for women with pelvic floor disorders needed improvement and cared enough to make it happen. Thank you to all the doctors who have decided to take on years of additional training to become certified in Female Pelvic Medicine and Reconstructive Surgery. Your expertise makes a huge difference for us as patients. Thank you to every doctor who has tried to make sense of pelvic floor disorders through rigorous experimentation and published research.

On a more personal note, thank you, Jon, for being my partner for the last ten years. For reading my first draft of this book and responding with compassion. For never asking me to omit a single word, though I describe some of our most difficult and personal shared experiences. As we used to say following disagreements, "I love you, I'm with you, and that's that." I am excited to move on from here with you.

Thank you to my postdoc advisor, Marla Feller, for encouraging me to take three months of maternity leave instead of the usual six weeks after my first child was born. You never knew how needed that was. I appreciated having those extra weeks to heal and adjust to my new reality. We need government-supported maternity leave policies in the United States, but that is a whole different book.

Thank you to my friends for showing up for me in big ways once I became bold enough to share what was really going on with my body. I love you.

Thank you to my mother, and to all the mothers, for making the world go round. I see you. You are stronger and more resilient than anyone gives you credit for, and you deserve to be treated with respect.

CHAPTER 1

"YOU ARE NOT MAKING UP THIS PROBLEM"

Seven years passed between the day I first noticed a strange bulge protruding out of my vagina and the day a doctor definitively told me what was going on with my body. If you are reading this book, I imagine you might be desperately seeking information you have been unable to find elsewhere, and so, I will begin near the end of my story. I will begin with answers.

If you leak urine, you have urinary incontinence. If you leak feces, you have fecal incontinence. If you have a bulge of tissue that protrudes out of your vaginal opening, you have pelvic organ prolapse. Urinary incontinence, fecal incontinence, and pelvic organ prolapse are the three primary pelvic floor disorders.

The most touted fix for pelvic floor disorders are Kegels, which are essentially strength training exercises for pelvic floor muscles. Try doing a Kegel right now. Place your hand over your crotch. Try to contract only the muscles below your hand, squeezing and lifting your crotch up. Not sure if you are doing it right? Next time you urinate, contract your muscles to stop the flow of urine. That is a Kegel.

Were you unable to stop the flow of urine with a Kegel? Were you unable to feel much of a contraction at all? If you answered yes to either or both of these questions, you are not alone. It may be that muscle weakness isn't your problem. It may be that your pelvic floor muscles and connective tissues have torn away from their anchor points. No amount of strength training can fix that.

Unfortunately for about 40% of women who leak urine and nearly all women who leak feces or have organs protruding from their vagina, Kegels are not going to fix their problems. Why? Pelvic floor trauma, such as the damage that occurs during vaginal childbirth, is the instigating cause of pelvic floor disorders. For many women the pelvic floor is damaged beyond what can be strengthened through exercise.

I am not saying that Kegels are worthless and you should not do them. Read Chapter 5 to learn the potential benefits of doing Kegels. I am saying Kegels are not enough. Women with pelvic floor disorders need more comprehensive care.

I got my answers from a doctor who completed extra training to become board certified in Female Pelvic Medicine and Reconstructive Surgery, earning the title of Urogynecologist. He is one of the heroes of my story. If your primary care or women's health doctor is shrugging off incontinence or prolapse as a normal part of the post-partum or aging experience, ask to be referred to a urogynecologist.

My urogynecologist's first sentence to me after his initial assessment was, "You are not making up this problem." Anyone who has struggled to get her pelvic floor disorder taken seriously will understand how comforting these words are.

Pelvic floor disorders are common, and their prevalence increases with age. In the United States, 6% of women develop at least one pelvic floor disorder between ages 20–29 years. This percentage increases incrementally with age and peaks at 53% in women aged 80 or older.[4]

The greatest risk factors for developing a pelvic floor disorder are giving birth and aging, though some women develop a pelvic floor disorder without ever having given birth, and some women develop one at a young age.

Pelvic floor disorders are embarrassing, and many women do not report their issues to their doctors. Even fewer women seek medical help for their pelvic floor disorders in developing countries, though they tend to have more children and are therefore at higher risk. In eastern Ethiopia, only 32% of women with pelvic floor disorders reported their concerns to a doctor.[5] Higher income and symptom severity were the best predictors of whether an individual sought medical care.

Prevalence numbers vary depending on what study you look at. The percentage of women with each pelvic floor disorder is determined by asking women to complete a questionnaire about their pelvic health. In some studies, diagnosis was confirmed with a gynecological exam.

In the United States, 17% of adult women had urinary incontinence, 9% fecal incontinence, and 3% pelvic organ prolapse.[4]

In rural Nepal, 24% of adult women had urinary incontinence, fecal incontinence was not assessed, and 8% had pelvic organ prolapse.[6] Most Nepalese women had 3 or more children *(range 1-15)*, so it makes sense that the prevalence of pelvic floor disorders was higher in Nepal than in the United States, where most women had fewer than 3 children.

In Tabriz, Iran, 50% of menopausal women had urinary incontinence, 16% fecal incontinence, and 55% pelvic organ prolapse.[7] In this case, diagnosis was confirmed with a gynecological exam. As in rural Nepal, the Iranian women typically had more than 3 children. This study also specifically looked at an older age group. These factors can explain the higher prevalence numbers here.

In urban Xi'an City, China, 23% of adult women had at least one pelvic floor disorder.[8] As in Iran, diagnosis was confirmed with a gynecological exam.

Pelvic floor disorders are clearly a significant health problem for women worldwide. Even taking the lowest reported values,

33% of women will have at least one pelvic floor disorder by age 55.[4]

This is a major women's health issue, and how many women have even heard of it? I hadn't. How can you know what symptoms to watch for and report to your doctor if you don't even know the words to use?

Reading this book will arm you with the language to use and the questions to ask when speaking with medical professionals. The more knowledge you have, the better you will be able to ask for what you need. In some cases, what you need is a second opinion from someone trained in Female Pelvic Medicine who will take your concerns seriously.

ANATOMY

It is important to learn the anatomy and function of the female pelvis to understand the cause of pelvic floor disorders and how they are treated. I will introduce the key players in pelvic floor disorders here. Please see Appendix A for more detail and additional illustrations. If you are more of a visual learner, you can find videos about female pelvis anatomy on my youtube channel.

Let's start with what we are all most familiar with: our external genitalia. Between our legs we can easily see our vulva and anus. Spreading the vulva apart, we can also see the clitoral hood, urethra, and vagina. The urethra, vagina, and anus have openings between the inside and outside of our bodies. These openings are normally held shut by contraction of the muscles that surround them. Pelvic floor disorders result from damage to the muscles, connective tissue, and nerves that work in concert to keep our urethra, vagina, and anus shut.

Each of our three pelvic openings has rings of muscle, called sphincters, around them. The sphincters are further supported by the levator ani muscles, which form the muscular bowl of the pelvic floor. If the sphincters or levator ani muscles become damaged, things you would rather keep on the inside, such as urine, feces, or your organs, make their way out without your permission.

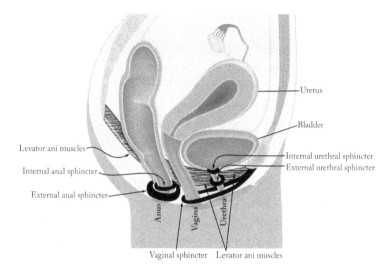

Each of our three openings is held shut by the combined action of sphincters and the levator ani muscles. For a more detailed look at the bands of levator ani muscles and how they contribute to continence and organ support, see Appendix A.

Of all the pelvic floor muscles, the levator ani muscles are the most valuable player, integrating and supporting all the rest. As mentioned, the levator ani muscles form the main bowl, or diaphragm, of the pelvic floor. Like the muscular diaphragm beneath our lungs, the pelvic diaphragm responsively supports the pelvic organs while we engage in everyday activities.

There is an additional layer of pelvic floor muscles, called the superficial layer, located between the levator ani muscles and the skin. The vaginal sphincter *(also known as the bulbospongiosus)* is one of the superficial muscles *(see above and Appendix A)*.

Each band of muscle is strung like a hammock between two attachment points. The central node of attachment for the superficial pelvic floor muscles is located between the vagina and the anus. Externally, the area between these openings is called the perineum. Beneath the skin of the perineum is the central node, called the perineal body *(also known as the central tendon of the perineum, see Appendix A)*. The perineal body is critical for the strength and integrity of the pelvic floor.

It can be helpful to think of the perineal body as a tent pole with many strings *(muscles)* tied to it. The strings extend outward in all directions from the tent pole, each going to its own second attachment point. Balanced tension on the strings is needed for the pelvic floor to do its job.

You can feel your own perineal body by making a thumbs up sign, sticking your thumb into your vagina so that it faces backward, and then pinching the perineum between thumb *(internal)* and forefinger *(external)*. If intact, your perineal body will feel thick with muscle. Keep your thumb in there and try doing a Kegel. Contract and lift your pelvic floor muscles up, toward your head. You should feel the perineal body lift inward while the muscles surrounding your vagina grip onto your inserted thumb. Ideally a Kegel will close the vaginal opening. There are three arches of muscle gripping your thumb and closing the vagina: the vaginal sphincter *(bulbosongiosus)*, the urethrovaginal sphincter *(an extension from the external urethral sphincter)*, and the pubovaginalis band of the levator ani muscles.

The vagina is the center of the pelvic universe. The locations of other organs are described relative to the location of the vagina. Anterior to *(in front of)* the vagina, we have the bladder. Posterior to *(in back of)* the vagina, we have the rectum. Apical to *(above)* the vagina, we have the uterus. In most women, the uterus tips forward and rests on top of the bladder.

Extending from the organs are sheets of connective tissue called fascia that attach to the side walls of the pelvis. Fascia act as walls to hold our organs in place.

The vagina and uterus are suspended above a gap in our pelvic floor muscles — the urogenital hiatus — with another type of connective tissue called ligaments. Ligaments act as weight-bearing ropes that hold our uterus and vagina up, keeping them clear of the urogenital hiatus. To describe how muscle and connective tissues work in concert, DeLancey wrote:

> "The longest-running debate [...] concerns whether muscle or connective tissue is the most critical element in pelvic organ support. Modern biomechanical analysis has shown that asking this question is like trying to decide which blade of a pair of scissors is the most important. The muscles and connective tissues involved in maintaining the pelvic organs in their normal locations act together to provide support in much the same way that the ventricles and valves are both needed for the heart to propel blood forward." [15]

The urogenital hiatus is our weak spot, because the levator ani muscles are not continuous there. If our levator ani muscles are a bowl, then the urogenital hiatus is an unsealed hole in the bowl. We must have this opening for intercourse and childbirth, but it comes at a cost.

When working properly, the levator ani muscles contract to close the urogenital hiatus and provide a lifting force as needed to cushion the organs and block their descent. In young, uninjured women, the levator ani muscles perform these functions automatically during daily activities. In fact, the only time uninjured women need to think about pelvic floor muscles at all is when they sit on the toilet, where they must relax their sphincters to let pee or poop out. If the levator ani muscles are injured such that they can no longer close the urogenital hiatus, incontinence and prolapse results.

The daily functions of the female pelvis are already demanding enough that our pelvic tissues can fail with age alone. Add to that the demands of pregnancy and vaginal childbirth, and the chances of failure increase greatly.

During pregnancy, the uterus grows in volume by more than 100 times, from 40 milliliters *(a shot of tequila)* to 4500 milliliters *(a gallon of milk)*.[9,10] The additional size and weight of the uterus puts pressure on the bladder, rectum, and pelvic floor.

The uterus connects to the vagina through a specialized fibromuscular neck of tissue called the cervix. The cervix terminates in the vagina, a muscular tube that opens to the outside world. The vagina is remarkably elastic and resilient. It is made of smooth muscle, collagen, and elastin fibers and has many folds called rugae so that it can expand.

During vaginal childbirth, the cervix, vagina, and urogenital hiatus must open to the size of the child's head circumference, typically between 31–39 centimeters.[11] For comparison, the circumference of a big *(29 oz)* can of black beans is 32 centimeters, and the circumference of the average adult woman's neck is 34 centimeters.

If the pelvic tissues cannot stretch wide enough, they tear. In some cases, the muscles and fascia rip away from their anchor points. This is called avulsion. One of the most common sites of tearing during vaginal delivery is along the arcus tendineus *(see Appendix A)*. Another is the perineum.

It is no surprise, then, that women who sustain severe pelvic floor trauma during vaginal delivery may have symptomatic pelvic floor disorders shortly following the birth of their first child. After having their first child, 12% of women report urinary incontinence, 10% report fecal incontinence, and 1.5% report pelvic organ prolapse.[4]

Women who have vaginal deliveries are much more likely to develop pelvic floor disorders, whether immediately after their first birth or several decades later. The current interpretation is that vaginal delivery damages the muscles and connective tissues of the pelvic floor but can take time to become symptomatic.

As women age and go through menopause the pelvic floor weakens further. The levator ani muscles become stiff and have diminished contractile and load bearing capacity.[12] Connective tissues become less elastic as estrogen levels go down.[13] If the pelvic floor was already weakened by vaginal delivery, symptoms of pelvic floor disorders are likely to start showing up at this time.

An estimated 78.84 million women worldwide have a spontaneous vaginal birth <u>each year</u>.[14] 26 million of them will develop at least one pelvic floor disorder by the time they are 65.

DIAGNOSIS

If you have symptoms of incontinence or notice an uncomfortable bulge in your vagina, it is important to report those problems to your doctor. Ask to be referred to a urogynecologist. If you live in a region of the world where there are no practicing urogynecologists nearby, ask to be referred to a doctor who specializes in pelvic health and has done surgical repairs for pelvic floor disorders. Your urogynecologist or specialist will then evaluate your pelvic floor and discuss treatment options.

I met with a urogynecologist seven years after the birth of my first child. To assess my pelvic health, he did an external and internal exam, followed by a bladder test.

I undressed from the waist down and lay on my back, knees bent. He asked me to cough a few times and watched my bulging tissues bulge out further. Then he did an external exam, pressing on different parts of my vulva and asking if I felt pain. He did an internal exam, inserting a gloved, lubed finger into my vagina and pressing onto each pelvic floor muscle. He inserted a speculum, had me cough a few more times, and took some measurements. Though I didn't feel much pain during the exam, I did feel pain afterward on the perineal side of my vaginal opening and told him so.

For the bladder test, he put a catheter inside my urethra, attached a conical vial, then backfilled my bladder with sterile water. He added water until I told him I felt like I needed to pee, then added more until I said I felt like I urgently needed to pee. Then he asked me to cough. Water squirted out. The test confirmed that I have urinary stress incontinence. Altogether these examinations took maybe 20 minutes.

Afterward I got dressed and we met in his office to discuss what he saw. He told me that I had three separate problems: pelvic organ prolapse, urinary incontinence, and vestibulodynia. We talked through the cause and treatment options for each disorder. I will introduce them here, along with fecal incontinence.

PELVIC ORGAN PROLAPSE

Pelvic organ prolapse occurs when the organs in your pelvis — the bladder, uterus, and rectum *(and, in rare cases, the small intestine or urethra)* — drop from their normal positions and invade the space normally occupied by your vagina *(see Appendix B for illustrations)*. Women with prolapse can see and feel a bulge or their cervix falling out of their body. They describe the feeling as one of heaviness, numbness, or pressure in their lower abdomen, vulva, and/or perineum.

Organs are held in place by membranous tissues. A defect in the membrane such as a weakness or a tear allows the organ to bulge out of its compartment. This is called a hernia. Prolapse of the bladder or rectum can be thought of as a hernia.

If the membranous fascia that normally creates a wall between the vagina and the bladder is damaged, the bladder can bulge through the hole in the wall. To be clear, the vagina itself remains intact, so what you observe is the anterior vaginal wall bulging in and down. The same thing can happen to the fascia between the vagina and the rectum. This would be observed as the posterior vaginal wall bulging in and down.

Prolapse of the uterus is a bit different. The cervix of the uterus already terminates in the vagina. It is suspended by ligaments. After pregnancy and childbirth, if the ligaments remain stretched out as the uterus shrinks down to its normal size, the uterus will drop down into the vagina. In this case, you would see your cervix either hanging low in the vagina or protruding out of it.

It has become standard to use POP-Q staging to quantify the degree of prolapse. Prolapse is symptomatic at POP-Q stage II or higher because the organs are low enough to push the urogenital hiatus open, blocking the closing and lifting support of the levator ani muscles.

POP-Q stages:

- Stage 0 is no organ descent.

- Stage I prolapse is bulge or cervix descent that has not reached the vaginal opening.

- Stage II prolapse is bulge or cervix descent to plus or minus one centimenter of the vaginal opening.

- Stage III prolapse is bulge or cervix descent of greater than 1 centimeter beyond the vaginal opening but less than the total vaginal length minus 2 centimeters.

- Stage IV prolapse is complete vaginal eversion, with organs descending as far as they can within the confines of the everted vagina.

My doctor told me I certainly had prolapse of the uterus and bladder, and I probably also had prolapse of the rectum, which he could assess better during surgery. Bladder prolapse is called anterior prolapse, since the bladder is in the anterior compartment of the pelvis and bulges into the anterior vaginal wall. It was formerly called cystocele. Similarly, rectal prolapse is called posterior prolapse, formerly rectocele.

For all types of prolapse, the only curative option is surgery. However, physical therapy can be effective in reducing some of your symptoms. I will discuss this further in Chapter 5. In addition, a pessary is a soft, flexible device that can be inserted into the vagina to provide structural support for your pelvic organs. Pessaries can reduce discomfort and manage symptoms in women who do not want surgery. I will discuss pessaries further in Chapter 6.

Behavior changes can also help with symptoms. Pelvic organ prolapse can cause problems with urine retention and constipation, since urine and feces can get "stuck" in prolapsed bladder or rectum resting below the urethral or anal openings *(Appendix B)*. Pelvic organ prolapse can also cause a feelings of numbness or discomfort when sitting or standing for long periods of time. There are tricks you can use to reduce these symptoms *(see Appendix C)*.

URINARY INCONTINENCE

Urinary incontinence is the involuntary release of urine. There are several types of urinary incontinence. Stress incontinence occurs when mechanical stressors to the bladder, such as coughing or jumping, cause some urine to leak out. Stress incontinence is the most common pelvic floor disorder among new mothers. Urgency incontinence occurs when the bladder detrusor muscle becomes overactive and squeezes urine out before you make it to the toilet. Overflow incontinence occurs when the bladder detrusor muscle is too weak to completely empty the bladder, which can result in leakage of retained urine. Anterior prolapse increases the likelihood of urinary retention, because a low sitting bladder requires a much stronger contraction to push urine up and out.

We have two sphincters around the urethra that cinch it shut to stop urine flow. The internal urethral sphincter is located at the point where the bladder meets the urethra. It is under involuntary control through the pudendal nerve.

A bit further down the urethra is the external urethral sphincter *(also known as the urogenital sphincter in women)*. It is under voluntary control. In females, the external urethral sphincter is a complex structure with three parts.

First is the proper urethral sphincter that forms a muscular ring around the urethra. As long as the external sphincter is constricted urine should not flow out, even if the internal sphincter is relaxed.

Second is the compressor urethral muscle that extends from either side of the ring and attaches to bone. This serves to lift and stabilize the urethra.

Third is a thin, broad muscle that encircles both the urethra and the vagina *(called the urethrovaginal sphincter)*. Contraction of this muscle constricts both the urethra and vagina. Collectively, the the external urethral sphincter is the muscle that stops urine flow when you do a Kegel.

Have you been counting? There are two sphincters dedicated to the urethra. In addition, there are three arches of muscle that encircle both the urethra and vagina. From the outside in, they are the vaginal sphincter *(bulbosongiosus)*, part of the external urethral sphincter *(urethrovaginal sphincter)*, and a band of the levator ani muscles *(pubovaginalis)*. These muscles work together to control the constriction of the urethra and urogenital hiatus.

As you can guess from this description of all the complex control mechanisms of urination, there are many ways this system can go wrong. Weak or torn sphincters, weak or torn levator ani muscles, or damage to the nerves that control these parts can all interfere with bladder control.

One outcome of weakened pelvic muscles and connective tissues is descent of the bladder neck. The bladder neck is the muscular tube surrounding the urethra between the bladder and the urethral opening. It is common for the bladder neck to descend after giving birth, tilting downward slightly. It is also common for the bladder neck to have increased mobility, where certain actions, like coughing or jumping, cause the bladder neck to descend even further, allowing urine to spill out like water from a tipped tea kettle.

Physical therapy *(i.e. Kegels)* improves control of urine flow in most women with stress incontinence. I will discuss that further in Chapter 5. However, if the bladder neck is tilted far down, the sphincter or levator ani muscles are severely damaged, or the fascia is torn causing anterior prolapse, surgical repair may be needed to stop leaking. A commonly used surgery to correct urinary incontinence is the placement of a mesh sling under the urethra. This holds up the bladder neck so urine is less likely to spill out.

If nerve damage is the culprit, one treatment option to try is nerve stimulation. Nerve stimulation encourages regeneration of the pudendal nerve and reinnervation of its targets in the pelvis, which reduces incontinence in some women. Urgency incontinence can be reduced through behavior changes or medication *(see Appendix C)*.

FECAL INCONTINENCE

Though I did not have issues with fecal incontinence and cannot share what that experience is like from a personal perspective, I include what I have learned from the medical literature here and throughout the book.

Fecal incontinence is the involuntary release of feces. Severe damage to the anal sphincters, as occurs with a 3rd or 4th degree vaginal tear during childbirth, can cause fecal incontinence. This degree of tearing is more likely if your obstetrician uses forceps to aid delivery. One study found that 53% of women who suffered a third degree vaginal tear developed fecal incontinence even though their tear was surgically repaired immediately following delivery.[16]

Weakened or torn levator ani muscles can also contribute to fecal incontinence. The puborectalis, a band of the levator ani, forms a sling around the rectum *(Appendix A)*. It holds the rectum at an angle, preventing the passage of stool to the anus. If this muscle weakens, incontinence may result.

As with urination, two sphincters control the release of feces. The internal anal sphincter is under involuntary control through the pudendal nerve. The external anal sphincter and the puborectalis muscle are under voluntary control and must relax to allow the passage of feces out of the rectum.

Though surgery does not have a high success rate as a long-term cure for fecal incontinence, there are many treatments to try. These include physical therapy with biofeedback, medications, and nerve stimulation techniques. I will discuss biofeedback and nerve stimulation in Chapter 5. There are also some simple behavior changes that can significantly improve symptoms for some women *(see Appendix C)*.

If fecal incontinence is your primary concern, you have two options for knowledgeable specialists. Ask to be referred to a urogynecologist or a colorectal surgeon.

VESTIBULODYNIA

Vestibulodynia, formerly called vulvar vestibulitis, is provoked pain and inflammation of the vulva. It can be triggered by the application of pressure or during vaginal penetration (intercourse or even a gynecological exam), sitting for long periods of time, or wearing tight-fitting pants.

Vestibulodynia is one of several disorders and allergic reactions that cause chronic pelvic pain, whether or not you have ever had children. Although it is not one of the three pelvic floor disorders, I am including it here because I imagine it is a common problem among women with pelvic floor disorders. I had this problem and it disproportionately contributed to my diminished quality of life. I also believe that my perineal damage and prolapse possibly caused, and definitely exacerbated, my vestibulodynia.

The pain from vestibulodynia is experienced differently by different women. It can be local or widespread. It can last for hours or days. Vestibulodynia can be caused by yeast, skin irritation, and/or nerve damage. A specialist assessment is necessary to identify the cause for each individual.

There is a surgical option called vestibulectomy to treat this problem, but this is rarely required.[17] Symptoms typically resolve without invasive treatments. My doctor prescribed 5% lidocaine ointment for the onset of vulvar pain following sex and a strong topical steroid ointment called clobetasol propionate to treat my chronic inflammation *(please note: topical steroids are intended for short-term treatment of inflammation followed by tapering off, and may cause problems if used daily for a long period of time).*

Importantly, he also gave me instructions for behavior changes, including hypoallergenic vulvar care *(see Appendix C).* Another common source of vulvar irritation and pain is shaving the pubic hair. So, trim it if you like, but think twice before you shave it off.

SURGICAL PLAN

DeLancey wrote, "Sadly, up to 1 of 5 women have pelvic floor disorders so severe that they require surgery during their lifetime for injuries largely attributable to changes resulting from birth."[3] Sadly, I was one of them.

Once my conditions were explained, my urogynecologist and I discussed treatment options including a surgical plan. I would get a hysterectomy, uterosacral ligament suspension of my vagina, anterior and posterior prolapse repair including possible tissue grafts with cadaver skin, and a urethra sling. These procedures are described in detail in Chapter 8.

The surgery would be long, estimated at 4–5 hours, but I was expected to go home the same day. The recovery would be long as well. At least one week lying in bed taking pain pills. Four weeks until I could bathe or swim or pick up anything heavier than ten pounds. Six weeks until I could have sex or engage in light exercise beyond walking. Twelve weeks until I could do whatever I wanted.

Neither of us anticipated that I had another, unseen problem that would require an additional surgical repair. This surprise resulted in a longer and more painful recovery.

Having a hysterectomy means you will not be able to have more children. Even if a hysterectomy is not in your surgical plan, it is best to wait until you are done having children before getting surgery to correct pelvic floor disorders. Otherwise you put yourself at risk of developing the same problems again, requiring a second surgical repair. These are serious surgeries. You do not want to put yourself through this more than once if you can help it.

My doctor advised that if my quality of life was not greatly affected by my condition, I should wait to get the surgery as long as possible. By the time I got to him I could no longer pee or poop without using my hand and fingers to assist, urine would sometimes flood out without warning and beyond the capacity of any pad, exercising exacerbated my symptoms, and sex led to days or weeks of an inflamed, painful vulva. I didn't want to wait anymore. With my go ahead, we started planning for surgery.

Now that you know where my story leads, let me tell you how I got there. It begins with the largest risk factor for developing pelvic floor disorders — giving birth.

CHAPTER 2

"THE NEXT ONE WILL FALL RIGHT OUT"

The day my eldest child was born was one of the happiest days of my life. I opted for an unmedicated labor and delivery in a hospital setting, with my husband by my side. My labor proceeded in textbook fashion for a first child. The first stage of labor, from the start of labor until the cervix dilates to ten centimeters, lasted about twelve hours. It hurt, but I knew the pain would end, and I would get to meet my baby girl.

My decision to turn down an epidural came from two beliefs. First, I believed it was important for me to experience what it feels like to give birth. I thought of it as a rite of passage and a shared experience that would connect me to my mother and all women throughout history. Second, I believed that my pain would guide me, helping me to cause less damage to my body.

Being in a hospital made it harder to stick to the "natural" birth plan. It has become a rarity for women in first-world countries to give birth without pain relief. In 2015, 71% of laboring women in the United States had an epidural or other spinal anesthesia.[18] There are certain variables, such as location, provider, and whether or not an individual has given birth before that further increase the odds of pain medication use.

A 2016 survey of 1,799 Californian women who had vaginal births reported that 77% of them used some type of pain medication.[19] Women who used an obstetrician or who were having their first child were the most likely to use pain medication.

I was offered drugs many times, requiring me to make my decision many times while in pain. As I entered transition, those last three centimeters of cervical dilation driven by the most intense contractions of labor, my doctor checked in to tell me that labor was about to get a lot more painful. She asked once again if I wanted any pain relief. I declined my last chance to get an epidural.

I knelt on the bed, facing the raised back and leaning on it for support. The contractions did hurt. I responded aggressively, gripping the bed and yelling. It felt good to be aggressive. Thankfully, the breaks between contractions were peaceful, enough so that I slept in those one-minute increments. I remember thinking how awful it felt during each contraction, but I couldn't speak. In between I felt completely fine and was able to rest.

The nurse told me that the baby would not drop if I kept clenching up during contractions and suggested that I lie back and focus on slow deep breathing, visualizing my body opening. I found that this strategy was much more painful, but labor progressed rapidly after this.

To anyone reading this who has not given birth, the closest experience I can think of for comparison is gastroenteritis. Uterine contractions feel a bit like the rolling stomach contractions that occur just before you involuntarily expel your stomach and/or intestinal contents, just far more intense. Both uterine and stomach contractions cause full body effects and an altered state of consciousness. They are not in our control. They are happening whether we want them to or not, though tension and fear can inhibit them from producing their intended result for a while.

The nurse said it wouldn't be much longer until it was time to push and predicted that I would be ready in another 30 minutes. My experience of time slowed at this point. There was a clock directly in my line of sight and a chart of cervix dilation. By my side, a device measured my uterine contractions. I remember staring in anger at these objects. Willing time to move forward. Willing my cervix to open to that absurd size of ten centimeters on the chart. Feeling anger and disbelief when only five minutes had passed in what felt like an hour.

During contractions, I watched the value of my muscle activity, waiting for it to drop so I could feel relief. I tried not to look at these things — the clock, the cervix diagram, the contraction sensor — but I could not stop. It was like running on a treadmill when you are nearing the end of your predetermined distance. You start to check the mileage obsessively, eagerly anticipating the end.

Finally, I started to feel like my girl was making her way down. At 2:40 pm the nurse told me it was time to start pushing. I remember being relieved and eager to push.

The second stage of labor, from ten centimeters dilated until the baby is delivered, lasted ninety minutes. The bed was made flat and the nurses prompted me to bear down with each contraction. Pushing felt good to me. I liked feeling that I had some degree of control, unlike uterine contractions. It was a purposeful, muscular effort. It also felt familiar, like engaging in an intense core strengthening workout.

During my second push, the amniotic sack broke and fluid shot across the room. I remember how satisfying that felt.

There was a shift change and a new nurse came along with a few additional nurses. They told me the doctor was busy delivering another baby. They set everything up for delivery. A warming table. Various tools. A mirror positioned so I could see what was happening. They did not have the same unclenched, deep breathing plan of my previous nurse.

I lay on my back, my husband holding one leg at the knee and my new nurse holding my other leg. I pushed. I stared at the clock. I got mad at the doctor. Almost thirty minutes passed before the doctor arrived. She geared up and sat at the end of the bed, headlamp on and gloved hands raised, as I pushed.

Pushing felt good, but the time between contractions did not, especially once my daughter's head started to make its exit. This is what they call the ring of fire, which is a beautiful way of describing the horrifying reality that your tissues are ripping apart.

As the child's head makes its way down the birth canal, it stretches the pelvic and vulvar tissues to the size of the child's head. Of course, you might think. And, of course, I knew that going in. What I didn't understand is that the head can be stuck there for a long time. In my case, my daughter's head was stuck in my vagina for over an hour. She was trapped because my labia and perineum were not stretchy enough to allow her exit. She had to rip her way out.

Between contractions, my doctor would insert lubed fingers between my perineum and my daughter's head and push against my perineum in a sweeping motion, trying to loosen the seal. After twenty minutes of this she offered to give me an episiotomy, saying, "One little snip and she'll fall right out."

I declined, so we continued our routine. I remained in this loop — feeling the contraction start up, pushing, seeing my daughter's dark matted hair pushing hard against my strained vulva, feeling the contraction subside and the ring of fire as she retreated back inside me, crying out in pain, feeling the doctor press down on my perineum, and repeat — for a full hour.

I told myself that every push was that last one. Just one more push, and I would get to see my daughter.

Finally, after my nurse coached me to do four intense pushes during a single contraction, my daughter crowned. It only took a few more contractions to get her out, and then there she was, lying on my chest.

I was euphoric. I felt no pain, only joy. My husband and I cried with joy. I don't remember feeling the afterbirth or the poking and prodding as the doctor stitched up my torn vagina and labia for an hour. My husband pulled a sheet over the three of us, creating a private tent, and we babbled at our baby girl with excitement. My daughter was awake and alert, not crying, staring at us as we told her again and again how happy we were to see her. We kept saying, "We have a baby! This is our baby! Hello, baby girl. We love you." As I said, even with all that pain, it was one of the best days of my life.

After I was stitched up, I sat up and breastfed her for the first time. It was only once she was taken away from me to be washed and measured that I realized how tired and sore and hungry I was. I still cannot fully process that a living human being developed inside of me and then my body opened wide enough to let her out. Giving birth is too fantastical to believe, even though it happens all the time. It is a biological miracle.

After my daughter was out, the nurse praised me for my strength and endurance. I felt proud. She asked if I was a long-distance runner. I said yes. Then she said, "The next one will fall right out." I remember thinking that would be nice, and wondering what that meant for my quality of life the rest of the time.

Never one to shy away from looking at my own private parts, it did not take long for me to notice that things weren't right. About a week after giving birth I noticed that a bulge of tissue was visible through my vaginal opening. At the perineal side of my vagina I could see my cervix. My thoughts as recorded in an email to a friend were, "I lost my vagina," "I think my uterus is falling out," and "My cervix is in the wrong place." I then called those thoughts ridiculous and wrote, "I am hoping that is all due to swelling and the slow retightening of muscles and ligaments and will magically fix itself."

Unfortunately, it never got better. What I was seeing was pelvic organ prolapse, but I had never heard of that at the time. The bulge was my bladder falling into my vagina through herniated connective tissue that normally separates the two. My uterus had fallen into my vagina as well, no longer held up by its ligaments that had been stretched beyond repair. As a result, my cervix was indeed much lower than it used to be. When lying down I had some relief and could feel that I did still have a vagina. But upon standing, my organs dropped in the direction of gravity, crowding my vagina with soft, fragile tissue. What was once a tight narrow muscular tube was effectively gone.

In hindsight, I have considered things I could have done differently that may have led to a different outcome. I read Ina May Gaskin's book on natural childbirth early in my pregnancy.[20] I understood the idea that giving birth requires opening a sphincter, like you do during a bowel movement. It is best not to strain, because straining may cause you to injure yourself. Instead, it is best to breathe deeply and release tension.

My nurses did not follow this approach. They repeatedly encouraged me to bear down and push as hard as I could. I was holding my breath and clenching my jaw with each push, so all the pressure was going into my pelvic floor. I dimly recalled that I wasn't supposed to and that straining causes damage, but I was in the worst pain of my life, and I wanted her out. Pushing felt good. It provided relief.

Perhaps if I had stuck to Ina May's approach I would not have torn so badly. Now I understand why people bring their own midwives or doulas to the hospital. If I had done so, the person in my ear would not have been pressuring me to push harder. They would have been helping me to breathe and relax and move into better positions so that my body could open wide enough to let my daughter pass.

Getting an epidural may have helped me reduce damage. Though counter intuitive to me at the time, feeling less pain would have made it easier to stick to an Ina May style delivery. I would not have needed the relief of muscular pushing.

Giving birth is a bodily trauma, and medical intervention can be a good thing. A review titled "Postpartum pelvic floor trauma," summarized that, "vaginal delivery results in direct

pelvic muscle trauma, disruption of fascial supports, and pudendal nerve injury." [21]

Damage to "fascial supports" can result in pelvic organ prolapse. Fifty percent of women have some degree of pelvic organ
prolapse after childbirth, with 10–20% developing symptomatic
prolapse *(prolapse that causes urinary, fecal, or sexual dysfunction)*
within their lifetime.[21]

Damage to pelvic muscles can cause urinary incontinence
or retention, fecal incontinence or constipation, and a range of
problems with sexual intercourse. 85% of women damage their
perineum during vaginal childbirth.[22] For most, this is a temporary discomfort that largely repairs with time. For the rest,
this is a permanent defect that can cause pain and disability. The
perineum is a central hub of attachment for fascia and multiple
bands of pelvic muscles. Even moderate injury to the perineum
can have a profound impact on quality of life.

The question of how to decrease damage to the pelvic floor
during vaginal childbirth does not have a clear answer. One
thing that is clear from the research is that operative vaginal
delivery, where forceps or a vacuum are used to assist delivery,
results in more damage than unassisted vaginal delivery. Every
study I looked at showed that women who had operative vaginal delivery had the worst outcomes. They had the most perineal damage and were far more likely to have problems with
fecal incontinence and sexual dysfunction.[23–25]

Another commonly used intervention is to give an episiotomy, purposefully cutting the perineum so that the baby can exit
without tearing perineal tissue. I wondered whether getting an
episiotomy would have saved me. However, episiotomy has not
proven to prevent pelvic floor disorders. Some studies show that
episiotomy increases the chances of developing one.[23]

My mom, who had short labors and unmedicated deliveries in hospitals, told me that the worst part of her recovery was
dealing with the pain from episiotomy. She told me to avoid
getting one if I could.

The instructor of my childbirth class in Berkeley, California also advised against episiotomy. She said the current medical consensus *(in 2012)* was that women heal better from a tear than from a cut. So, when the doctor offered me an episiotomy, I wrote her off as old school.

When recounting my birth story, I referred to my doctor as the devil on my shoulder, since she kept offering me tempting things that I said I didn't want. Maybe she was right, though. In some cases, an epidural, episiotomy, or Cesarean section *(C-section)* may be best. Perhaps she knew from experience that her intervention would have made my delivery less damaging. I wonder if that is what she was thinking about as she stitched up my tears.

Not too long ago it was common for women to die during childbirth. In 1918, 916 out of every 100,000 live births in the United States resulted in the death of the mother.[26] By 2018, the maternal mortality rate reduced to 17.4 out of every 100,000 births in the United States, and to just 3 out of 100,000 in Finland. Medical intervention during labor and delivery saves lives.

Unfortunately, the healthcare system in general and obstetricians in particular have lost the trust of the public when it comes to childbirth. The pervasive opinion is that money hungry or time-conscious doctors push unnecessary medical interventions onto laboring women.[27] Expectant mothers now come into the hospital with a birth plan, and doctors are not supposed to push back against those wishes unless the mother or child's life is in danger.

My doctor politely pushed back against my wishes, and I despised her for it. If she were anything but an obstetrician, I would have respected her authority as a doctor and let her guide me toward good decisions. In my mind, she was only there as a precautionary measure, in case me or my baby needed an intervention for our survival.

Part of the reason I didn't connect with my obstetrician is because I had never met her before. We only spoke while I was in labor pain. Having never met her before, it was all too easy to label the person pushing against my wishes as the enemy.

Obstetricians are not the enemy. They have experience and information that might help you to have the best possible outcome. The Guardian article, 'We know the reality of childbirth,' reports that 50% of female obstetricians in the United States would opt for a C-section for their own delivery.[28] Multiple studies have shown what obstetricians already know, that women are less likely to develop pelvic organ prolapse or fecal incontinence after C-section.[29-31]

The notion of opting for a C-section to avoid damage to the pelvic floor is highly controversial. C-sections can cause significant complications, resulting in disability or death in some cases, and may not entirely prevent the onset of pelvic floor disorders. The World Health Organization holds steady in their advice that a C-section rate of 10-15% is ideal.[32] That rate is based on the use of C-sections only in cases where the lives of the infant or mother are in danger. At C-section rates higher than 10%, infant and maternal mortality rates no longer decrease. Hospitals around the world already exceed this rate.

We can all agree that a C-section to save a life is a good choice. But what about protecting quality of life? Should C-sections be used for patients who are at high risk of pelvic floor disorders? That is less clear. It is also moot in 2020. There is currently no way to say with certainty whether an individual will sustain severe damage to her pelvic floor during delivery or what her individual risk of developing a pelvic floor disorder is.

Ideally, obstetrician gynecologists would be able to advise each individual on their mode of delivery during prenatal appointments. To get there, we need to understand what assessments can reliably predict when an individual is likely to sustain severe damage from vaginal delivery, and what the optimal preventative strategy is. I hope that with additional research, doctors will better understand the risk factors for pelvic floor disorders and develop multiple preventative strategies.

Whether or not preventative measures can be taken, women need to be educated about their pelvic floor during their first pregnancy. These conversations can happen with their obstetrician gynecologist and during childbirth classes.

Given the high chance of developing a pelvic floor disorder and the potential for severely degraded quality of life, every pregnant woman should be told that giving birth may result in damage to their pelvic floor tissues. They need to know what pelvic floor disorders are, what symptoms to look for, and when to seek medical attention.

I went into my postpartum check-up naive. I knew things were not right, but I didn't know that my problems could be permanent. I did not know the right words to use or questions to ask. Unfortunately for me, the doctor I saw for my postpartum checkup was not very knowledgeable about pelvic floor disorders either.

CHAPTER 3

"JUST HAVE MORE SEX"

B y the time of my six-week postpartum check-up my stitches had dissolved, and the swelling was gone, but the bulge was still there. My bladder had settled into my vagina, resting just above the opening. The bulge of tissue pushed my labia open slightly, giving me what doctors call a "gaping vagina." My cervix was also resting just above my vaginal opening. Both were visible to me when I sat on the toilet.

The bulge created pressure and discomfort, making ordinary movements feel unnatural and uncomfortable. I had enough urine leaking out that I needed to wear pads every day. I had a chronically inflamed, painful vulva. After a long day I would lie down and feel it throbbing. The pulsing pain turned into tissue irritation and hypersensitivity. Once triggered, the pain could last days or even weeks. Pinching my labia provided some pain relief but could also result in open sores, so I learned to apply ice instead.

It was with this devastating new normal in mind that I went to my six-week check-up. My doctor shrugged off my concerns. He told me to "just have more sex" to strengthen my pelvic floor muscles. He checked me for a yeast infection and found none.

He gave me a topical 1% hydrocortisone cream to apply to my inflamed vulva and sent me on my way.

Knowing what I know now, this completely unsatisfactory advice from my doctor is infuriating. At the time, I was happy to hear it. It made sense to me. It was a relief to think that things might still get better, and that something as simple and enjoyable as sex might fix it. The only problem with his advice in my mind was, how was I supposed to have a lot of sex with my broken, inflamed parts?

For me, great sex comes from those present being uninhibited and open to all types of intimate touch that create pleasure. There is a great deal of trust and comfort needed to fully engage in sexual activity. We trust that our partners accept us and want us. We trust that they will tell us if something we are doing is generating unpleasant sensations or emotions. We trust that they will listen to any discomfort we may have and adjust.

I broke that trust completely. I was embarrassed about the condition of my body and tried to keep it a secret from my husband for almost two years. 'How could that even be possible?' you might wonder. Well, I rejected his sexual advances a lot. Anytime my vulva was inflamed, which was often, I pushed him away with little to no explanation.

I could no longer have sex without embarrassment in any position but missionary, so I kept us stationary. As I mentioned, I had the semblance of a vagina while lying down. It was only when upright that the bulge was visible. Any position where I was upright caused discomfort and embarrassment. For example, when I was on top, the bulge would hang low. His penis would physically displace my organs with each thrust, creating suction and noise not unlike plunging a toilet.

In missionary position, my organs were not visibly bulging out of me, so I could keep my secret. It didn't feel the same, but it was the least noxious.

I used to easily have orgasms during vaginal penetration. For quite a while after childbirth, the overall sensation of sex was a dull numbness, plus the strange new feeling of my organs getting pushed around.

When I regained sensation my vulvar and vaginal sensory map had changed. I had more pain-triggering spots and less pleasure-inducing spots. This experience of a period of numbness followed by painful touch-sensation was likely due to the slow regeneration of sensory nerves that had been damaged during childbirth.

My clitoris was intact and still produced pleasure, but I often rejected or interrupted oral sex. When inflamed, my irritated vulva sometimes caused pain at the slightest touch. My vulva was often swollen and red. Between that and my gaping vagina I felt self-conscious about the appearance of my genitals.

It was difficult for me to feel much pleasure given these conditions, and that was obvious to my husband. Sometimes I would think that I was well enough to have sex, and then once we started, I could feel my tender parts starting to scream out in irritation. Rather than tell my husband what was going on, I would clench my muscles and try to push through it.

It wasn't quite as deceptive as it sounds, because I felt pleasure in addition to the pain. Sometimes the pleasure would win out and I might even orgasm. Sometimes the pain would win, and he would eventually give up. He is a giving sexual partner, a man who is most turned on by seeing and feeling his partner in a state of pleasure. My clenched non-responsive body was effectively a rejection, even though my mind didn't want to reject him.

The worst part was that I hurt afterward. Sex caused painful, itchy inflammation of my vulva that lasted for days or weeks afterward, so I rejected advances until I got that back under control.

Imagine how this would feel from his end. A lot of rejection with no explanation. He is not one to push through rejection and mistreatment and take me anyway. He stopped initiating sex or being affectionate with me at all. I stopped being intimate with him in other ways because I worried it would lead to him wanting sex and me having to hurt him with another rejection.

The result? A sexless marriage, defined as having sex less than ten times a year. A big part of what caused this was my reluctance to be honest with him about what was going on with my body. I thought this would be a temporary deceit. I thought sharing the problems I was having would be unsexy. You know what is more unsexy? Rejection. Loss of trust. Loss of physical intimacy in its entirety.

I was finally honest with my husband after accepting that it was not going to get better, but that didn't happen until years had passed. My temporary solution of hiding the truth from my husband was not so temporary.

I have always been a highly sexual person. I was in a nearly continuous series of monogamous, sexually active relationships since I was fourteen years old. I believe, and scientific evidence and common sense concur, that sex and orgasm have incredible physical and mental health benefits. After giving birth I could not imagine having sex and having it result in anything but pain.

I am hardly alone in this problem. As many as 64% of women experience some sort of sexual dysfunction in the first year after giving birth.[33] This includes dyspareunia *(painful sexual intercourse)*, sexual desire disorder, orgasmic problems, and sexual arousal disorder. In one study, 50% of women reported having dyspareunia six weeks after childbirth, with 40% still reporting it by six months.[34] In another study, 17% of women reported having dyspareunia one year after childbirth.[35]

Women are typically told that they can resume having sexual intercourse four to six weeks after giving birth. For women who sustained severe perineal trauma or damage to their sphincters during delivery, this short recovery period is insufficient. Healing takes time.

A recent study of sexual health found that although 73% of women had resumed sexual intercourse by six months after delivery, they had low sexual function scores. Women who had obstetric and sphincter injuries, which is severe trauma to the perineum, were less likely to have resumed sexual intercourse and had lower sexual function scores than those without injuries. In keeping with other studies, women who had operative vaginal deliveries *(forceps or vacuum assisted)* fared the worst. In comparison to women who had spontaneous deliveries, women who had operative deliveries were even less likely to have resumed having intercourse and had the lowest sexual function scores.[36]

One criticism I have of this study is that the question, "Have you resumed coital activity?" is insufficient without some sort of explicitly stated threshold. The answer to the question would be yes whether they are having sex once a month or once a day. I imagine most women, like me, want to resume having sex with their partners and try their best to do so, but are only able to infrequently. Asking something more specific, such as, "How many times did you have sexual intercourse in the last two weeks?" would be more informative. This is somewhat remedied by assessment of sexual function with a PISQ-12 questionnaire, but frequency of intercourse was not one of the 12 questions.

One reason why most women with severe injuries had resumed sexual intercourse by six months may be that pain from injury typically subsides by then. Though some women still experience pain during intercourse after a year, they are in the unlucky minority. The authors point to "a previous report of a gradual improvement of perineal pain from two to six months after delivery."[37] The decrease in pain by six months would make resumption of sexual intercourse more likely.

A 1987 study summarizes the typical time course of postpartum sexual activity as follows:

"Most research respondents reported gradual return to prepregnancy levels of sexual desire, enjoyment, and coital frequency, with a minority in most cited studies indicating sexual interest and coitus levels below prepregnancy levels up to 1 year after delivery. The most frequently listed reasons for poor postpartum sexual adjustment include episiotomy discomfort, fatigue, vaginal bleeding or discharge, dyspareunia, insufficient lubrication, fears of awakening the infant or not hearing him/her, fear of injury, and decreased sense of attractiveness. Postpartum counseling should be offered prior to hospital discharge." [38]

Unsurprisingly to me, multiple sexual health studies showed that women who were still breastfeeding at 6 months had lower sexual function scores. [36,39] Personally, I have never been more tired or sick of being touched as while breastfeeding a six to twelve-month old. In addition, breastfeeding lowers estrogen levels, which contributes to pain during intercourse. If you are breastfeeding and experiencing pain during intercourse, you can ask your doctor to prescribe a low dose vaginal estrogen cream to treat your pain.

Reviewing the medical literature, it looks like postpartum sexual function first started being studied in the 1980s, with 1-4 publications on the topic per year until 2000. Since then, the publication rate has been increasing, with an average of 28 publications per year over the last five years. Though these publications all report that sexual dysfunction and painful intercourse are likely for the first year after childbirth, it has not become common practice to ask women about their postpartum sexual function or provide counsel. Expecting couples should be told that sexual dysfunction is likely after childbirth and advised on ways to maintain intimacy.

My advice? Assume that vaginal penetration is off limits, unless the person who has given birth decides otherwise. Leave the breasts alone as well unless you have permission. Of women I have spoken to, most breastfeeding women do not want their breasts used for sexual intimacy during that time, especially during the first several months or so when breasts are tender. What is left? Plenty! Touching, massage, snuggling, kissing, mutual masturbation, and oral sex are all ways to be intimate that do not cause pain. Engage in these activities often, with no pressure to have them lead to intercourse.

If you do choose to have sexual intercourse, go slow and be honest. If it hurts, say so, stop what you are doing, and try something else. Use lube, even if you feel like you don't need it. If deep penetration triggers pain, you can try using a 'sex doughnut,' which is a soft silicone ring that is placed around the penis and pulled down to the base. It acts as a bumper so that the penis cannot go too deep into the vagina.

You may notice that there are certain sensitive spots in your vagina that trigger pain. It can be helpful to experiment and see what sexual positions might work best to avoid your sensitive spots.

Eventually, a physical therapist gave me a printout of "Orthopedic Considerations for Sexual Activity." [40] The document shows thirteen standard sexual positions and lists the advantages and potential pain caused by each one. If you are having problems with pain during intercourse, I recommend asking your doctor for a copy, or paying the $20 to purchase one. Alternatively, if you and your partner have good communication about sex, you can try different positions and identify the ones that result in the most pleasure and least pain.

For example, I wrote that I restricted myself and my partner to missionary position after giving birth to my first child because it was the least embarrassing for me. However, this position is listed as one that may be uncomfortable for women with anterior or uterine prolapse because it stimulates the anterior wall of the vagina. In my experience, it can also put a lot of pressure on the perineum, which is not great while recovering from a perineal tear or if you have vestibulodynia. In contrast, having the man enter from the rear when the woman is positioned in doggy style or a supported kneeling position will be less bothersome to women with anterior or uterine prolapse, but may be uncomfortable for women with posterior prolapse, since it stimulates the posterior vaginal wall. It is also a great position for manual stimulation of the woman's clitoris, perineum, or anus, and for caressing the woman's breasts, so if she has reduced sensation in and around her vagina she can receive pleasurable stimulation in many other ways. Indeed, after getting this advice *(unfortunately just a few months before I got my surgery)*, my sex life improved dramatically.

For women who are injured badly enough during childbirth to develop pelvic floor disorders immediately afterward, sexual dysfunction and pain during intercourse are almost guaranteed. This is just one of many ways that our quality of life is diminished.

CHAPTER 4

"DEGREE OF BOTHER"

My pelvic floor disorders had many negative effects on my quality of life. One, as just described in detail, was loss of sexual intimacy with my husband. Another big change was loss of exercise.

I have always been an active person. Long distance running has been my go-to favorite exercise since I was ten years old. Running now felt awful. The prolapse bulge would bounce up and down, putting more pressure on my labia, and urine would leak out continuously. Running made me feel like I had developed an unsightly, sensitive scrotum. I quit running.

I tried other forms of exercise. Walking was ok, so I took a lot of long walks with my daughter. Yoga was ok too, but only if I was alone, which was almost never at the time. Yoga has a lot of forward folds, leg lifts, and inverted poses. Transitioning into and out of those poses would cause vaginal flatus, a noisy uncontrolled rush of air out of my vagina. Not something you want to have happen in a yoga class.

I leaked urine all the time. The simple act of moving from a seated to standing position would cause some urine to spill out. To deal with this I started wearing incontinence pads every day. These are like a maxi pad, but are designed to absorb and neutralize the odor of urine. However, tissue that should be inside of me was now exposed to the outside through my gaping vagina. My tender mucosal tissue would rub on the pad, creating irritation. As a result of this and the pressure of the bulge, sitting or standing for a long time was painful.

I also had issues with urine retention and an overactive bladder. I returned to work three months after giving birth and found that I needed to develop strategies to make it through my day without too much urine leaking out. I would avoid drinking anything for a few hours prior to my departure. Even so I typically needed to duck into a coffee shop near my bus stop to urinate before walking the final ten minutes to the lab where I was a postdoctoral researcher at the time. I learned not to jostle my body too much. How to get off the bus gently. How to bend down to pick something up without pushing urine out. How to sit down and stand up while contracting my pelvic floor. How to exhale while lifting something heavy.

Put another way, my pelvic floor disorders changed the way I move in the world. I started to opt out of activities that I used to enjoy. Sex, exercise, social gatherings, work. All had the potential to create discomfort, pain, and embarrassment.

My physical disability and dramatic changes to my quality of life were hard to adjust to. Unsurprisingly, I started to feel depressed. Without adequate sleep, exercise, or physical intimacy to soothe me I sought comfort elsewhere. I turned to alcohol and called it self-care. I was definitely in the problem drinking category.[41] I would typically have three drinks a day, spread out over many hours. When in an especially depressed mood I might have four or five.

When my daughter grew old enough to say some words, she started to ask for sips of my alcoholic beverages. I told her that she couldn't drink it, because it was my medicine, and mommy needed her medicine.

Ironically, alcohol is a bladder irritant and can exacerbate urinary urgency and incontinence. More alcohol consumption always results in me drinking more coffee as well, another irritant. I was unwittingly making my symptoms worse.

My experience was similar to that of others with pelvic floor disorders. Researchers have assessed changes in quality of life through questionnaires, interviews, and analysis of conversations on message boards. These are considered subjective measures, because they depend on each individual self-reporting what it is like for them to have a pelvic floor disorder. No one outside of the afflicted person can validate or deny their personal experience.

This is in contrast to objective measurements, such as the distance an individual's prolapsed organs protrude outside the vaginal opening or the volume of urine leakage during a cough. Any person could make the same measurement and get the same value for a given individual.

Subjective measures must be taken seriously in medical research and when treating patients. The ultimate goal is for the patient to feel that they are healthy and symptom free.

Young or old, living in the United States, Saudi Arabia, China, South Africa, or Sweden, women with pelvic floor disorders have a shared list of ways their quality of life has been affected.[42–47] Commonly affected areas of life are sexual intimacy, physical activities, social interactions, and work. Honestly, what is left?

Depression is more prevalent among women with symptomatic pelvic floor disorders.[43,44,48,49] Women who experience pain or fecal incontinence during intercourse tend to report higher levels of depression.[50] Low genital self-image among women with pelvic floor disorders is also associated with low sexual function scores and high rates of depression.[51]

Many research papers on this subject reported that depression correlated to lower quality of life scores in women with pelvic floor disorders. However, quite a few studies interpreted this in a way that made me angry. For example, one study used a questionnaire that essentially asks, 'how much do your symptoms bother you?' *(the PFDI-20 questionnaire, included in Ap-*

pendix D). Women who indicated a higher level of bother also tended to be depressed *(both subjective measures)*, even though the objective measurements taken were not different between individuals. The author's conclusion was, "It may be that depressed patients interpret their symptoms differently." [52] This statement suggests that positive thinking would alleviate the impact of pelvic floor disorders.

A better interpretation, in my opinion, is that the daily experience of pain and disability caused by pelvic floor disorders, and the resulting diminished capacity to engage in work, friendships, intimate relationships, and exercise, makes depression more likely. In my opinion, this study also indicates that there are anatomical and physiological differences between women with the same objective measurements that were not detected by those measurements.

What objective measurements can be used to predict pelvic function or disability? From reading John O.L. DeLancey's research papers, I see that the anatomical indicators of disability are beginning to be elucidated.[15] One factor that significantly increases the severity of symptoms is functional loss of the levator ani muscles. This is caused by neurological and structural damage from the stretching and tearing of muscles away from their anchor points. When the levator ani muscles are damaged such that they no longer function there is a huge biomechanical impact. Basic functions such as peeing, pooping, and moving are all affected. DeLancey wrote that the threshold for disability is loss of 50% or more of the levator ani muscle and/or a decrease of 40% or more in levator ani muscle contractile strength.

Subjective measures have pulled out some interesting differences in the ways women experience having a pelvic floor disorder. Women who have symptomatic prolapse immediately following childbirth have a different experience than women who gradually develop prolapse as they age.[44,46]

Women who had to adapt to symptoms of pelvic organ prolapse while caring for a newborn had a lot more anger.[46] They felt that they were not adequately warned that this could happen, had a hard time getting accurate information about what was going on, and that their postnatal doctors trivialized their problems. As the authors put it, "The feeling of being taken by a dreadful surprise was prominent in the women's stories." Of all the research articles I read, this one was most like reading a diary of my experience. Here is their summary of results in full:

> "The overarching theme 'being irreparably damaged' was identified as representing an experience of being disabled by sPOP [symptomatic pelvic organ prolapse] after vaginal birth. The fertile women experienced that their lives were ruined because of physical and psychological limitations caused by this unexpected, unfamiliar, and unexplained condition. Living with sPOP impinged on sexual health, restricted daily and sports activities and affected the women's ability to fulfill everyday parental duties. This in turn compromised women's psychological health. In addition, the negligence of healthcare professionals who tended to trivialize and normalize the symptoms led to the belief that there were no sustainable treatments and that women would have to live with bothersome symptoms of POP for the rest of their lives."

Women who developed symptomatic pelvic organ prolapse over time were more likely to ruminate on how they were getting older and falling apart.[44] Elderly women often wait to seek treatment until their symptoms become severe, and may then find themselves talking to doctors who shrug off their pelvic floor disorders as a common part of aging. Common does not mean acceptable. If your concerns are ignored, ask to be referred to a urogynecologist.

Throughout the research literature, the age of 65 is arbitrarily used as the threshold of entering old age. It is important to recognize that there are many healthy, energetic women over the age of 65 who are still sexually active and who are still working, volunteering, traveling, and caring for grandchildren among other activities. All these activities are hindered by pelvic floor disorders. For women who have become frail or have decreased mobility due to other medical conditions, their pelvic floor disorders not only impact their lives but the lives of their caregivers, who must help them get to bathroom and clean up their accidents.[54]

These differences aside, the experience of dealing with pelvic floor disorders is largely shared between these two groups. The study of women who developed prolapse later in life found that, "The feeling of brokenness and incompleteness surfaced also in a discussion of how prolapse affected the participant's intimate relationships and how this made her feel. In a similar fashion, some described feelings of not being a whole woman." [44] The study of women with prolapse immediately after giving birth found that, "A nearly non-existent sex life resulted in feelings of being non-sexual, disabled and destroyed as a woman." [46]

In addition to shared devastation at the loss of sexual intimacy, women young and old shared each other's physical pain. "The women described feelings of constant discomfort which severely disrupted daily life, such as pressure, heaviness, fullness, and the sensation that something was falling out of the vagina. …This constant discomfort was compounded by basic day to day activities such as cooking and walking, and even standing or sitting." [46]

They also had similar fears. They feared worsening symptoms and were unsure of what preventative measures to take. They shared feelings of being alone in their problems, and had difficulty discussing them with partners or friends. "Alongside identifying pelvic floor disorders as taboo, some women identified a sense of shame that made talking about their symptoms even more challenging. Women described secrecy surrounding pelvic floor disorders even amongst other women." [44]

Perhaps the group of women who are most isolated are those with fecal incontinence. I am not sure why poop is such a taboo subject and source of embarrassment for women, but it certainly is. I know that out of all my symptoms, I have been most reluctant to share my problems with bowel movements, which became troublesome after my second child was born. My poop problems also crossed the line for me. It was at that point that my symptoms went from being bothersome to being intolerable. But my problems were with poop getting stuck inside me and were easy to keep secret. What if my poop started spontaneously and involuntarily coming out at inappropriate times, like having coffee with friends, on a run, and during intercourse?

As you might guess, fecal incontinence has a profound impact on quality of life. Women with fecal incontinence are likely to avoid intercourse and stop exercising. Some women with this problem worry so much about leaking that they quit their jobs and reject offers to socialize. As reported by The Guardian, colorectal surgeon Michelle Thornton said, "Most are too embarrassed to go out. They will not go anywhere unless they know there is going to be a toilet. They can't use public transport; they don't go out for meals . . . Only two of them have managed to keep a job, the rest don't because they think they smell all the time. If they cough or sneeze or laugh they know they are going to leak." [28]

Consider this excerpt from a review by Isuzu Meyer and Holly E Richter to see what it is like to have fecal incontinence *(FI)* on your mind.

> "For women with FI, going out or traveling causes great anxiety and much planning. Many women fast for hours or days as a strategy to avoid bowel leakage when they have to leave their house. The availability and accessibility of a restroom is a major concern. They are acutely aware of bowel control and are conscious of where the nearest toilets are when they are away from home. This process is known as 'toilet mapping' to reduce the risk of a bowel accident." [54]

It is no wonder that many of us experience depression and anxiety. About six months after my second child was born, I went through a depressive episode. My depression was caused in part by my worsening symptoms, which I will describe more in Chapter 6. I was in some serious denial, and the only way I got out of my depression and substance abuse cycle was to have my husband, a therapist, and a psychiatrist tell me that I was depressed and needed help within a few weeks of one another. Only then did I believe that I had a problem.

I was extremely reluctant to try antidepressants, after watching friends and family members struggle to find anything that helps them while dealing with the side effects of going on and off these medications. My psychiatrist patiently and persistently told me that antidepressants are far more specific and less damaging than alcohol.

I started taking an antidepressant and am still taking it now. It isn't an ace in the hole, but overall, my depression is less frequent and less severe. I was sober for 14 months. I have resumed drinking alcohol but make sure to keep my drinking within the recommended limits. The CDC recommendation for women is seven servings or less of alcohol a week, and never more than three servings in a day. Even with my depression largely cured and my alcohol use in check, I continued to experience a great deal of bother and diminished quality of life from my pelvic floor disorder symptoms, enough so that I sought surgery to correct my problems.

To others with substance abuse or depressive disorders, I strongly encourage discussing these problems with your doctor. If your doctor is not receptive, find a psychiatrist, join a support group, or talk to a friend. It is important to consider these issues seriously. That may mean you need to limit your interaction with people who normalize substance abuse behaviors.

Daily drinking habits have become a normalized behavior for affluent mothers of young children *(at least in the U.S.)*. For women with depressive tendencies, substance abuse is dangerous. Not only is it toxic for your body, it is likely to trigger a depressive episode. I would love to see women encouraging each other to make healthy choices, rather than normalizing unhealthy choices. If your friend expresses concerns about her substance use, listen. Don't make jokes and offer to buy the next round.

To any postnatal health care providers reading this, I strongly encourage you to inquire about your patient's substance use and depression symptoms, and then follow up with an appropriate treatment plan. Consider making the intervention approach used in the referenced study by Wilton DP et al. a new standard of postnatal care *(see* [53]*)*.

Though incontinence and prolapse are common, they should not be trivialized and treated as an inevitable consequence of giving birth or aging. For each pelvic floor disorder there are adjustments you can make to improve your quality of life and reduce the strain on your body as you explore treatment options. Some of them are listed in Appendix C.

This book is a good start, but it is essential that you push for more from your health care providers. Many women find that some of their primary care doctors and gynecologists are not very knowledgeable about pelvic floor disorders. Even if they are, they are unlikely to ask you unprompted questions about your urinary, bowel, prolapse, and sexual symptoms. Until standard obstetrics and gynecology protocols change, getting the help you need is up to you. If you are experiencing symptomatic pelvic floor disorders, talk to your doctor about them and ask to be referred to a urogynecologist.

CHAPTER 5

"HAVE YOU TRIED KEGELS?"

By far the most common question I received upon telling friends about my problems was, "Have you tried Kegels?" Yes. I have tried Kegels, thank you.

It wasn't just friends, though. Doctors and nurses also pushed the idea that physical therapy, i.e. Kegels, might improve my symptoms or even cure my pelvic floor disorders.

Where does this faith in the Kegel come from, and can they help with pelvic floor disorders?

Kegel exercises were first described in a scientific journal by Los Angeles based gynecologist Arnold Kegel *(1894-1972)*. Kegel intended his exercises to be used for the treatment of stress urinary incontinence.[55] In all of Kegel's papers, he points to vaginal childbirth as the cause of decreased pelvic floor muscle strength.

Many research papers validate this claim. In a paper published in 2013, researchers tested the pelvic floor muscle strength of 277 pregnant women throughout pregnancy and six weeks postpartum. The women who had C-sections had a

10% reduction in the resting tone of their pelvic floor muscles. In contrast, the women who had vaginal deliveries had a 29% decrease in resting tone as well as a 54% decrease in strength and a 53% decrease in endurance. Those who required the use of instruments such as forceps during delivery fared even worse, with 30% reduction in resting tone, 66% reduction in strength, and 65% reduction in endurance. Women who developed urinary incontinence after delivery had significantly weaker pelvic floor muscle strength and endurance than those who did not.[25]

My first attempt at Kegel exercises postpartum made me laugh, because my muscles were weak and my sensory nerves were shot. I couldn't feel any muscles contracting. Only by sticking my hand over my vaginal opening or my finger inside my vagina could I get the sensory feedback that I was slightly contracting my pelvic floor muscles when I tried to do a Kegel.

Kegel's first paper on the subject was published in 1948. His suggestions were largely ignored until the 1980s. Since then, there have been about one hundred medical studies on the efficacy of Kegel exercises for women with urinary incontinence.

Looking through the more recent research literature, it appears that Kegel exercises help most women to improve their stress urinary incontinence problems. A systematic review and meta-analysis of 31 trials found that 56% of women with stress urinary incontinence reported that their symptoms were cured and 74% cured or improved at the conclusion of physical therapy treatment.[56] The percent improvement appears to be similar whether exercises are done by postpartum or elderly populations.

The author's of one study noted, "An active voluntary pelvic floor muscle contraction before a sudden intra-abdominal pressure rise *('perineal lock' [AKA the Knack])* appeared to be responsible for most of the success." [57] As one demonstration of this, it has been found that elderly women with mild to moderate stress urinary incontinence can reduce urine leakage by 73-98% within just one week of being taught to contract their pelvic floor muscles during a cough.[58] The timing of the contraction proved more important than contractile strength.

A study titled "Pelvic Muscle Exercises: When Do They Work?" found that Kegels improved symptoms for 56% of their incontinent research subjects. However, they divided their women into three categories, mild, moderate, or severe urinary incontinence, based on objective measures. They found that women with severe stress incontinence were less likely to see an improvement in their symptoms.[59]

Most of these studies specifically assessed the effects of Kegel exercises on stress urinary incontinence. However, urinary incontinence can be caused by increases in intra-abdominal pressure *(stress)*, a sudden need to urinate immediately *(urgency)*, or dribbling of retained urine due to inefficient bladder emptying *(overflow)*. Some women are dealing with two or three types of incontinence. Will Kegels work for them? The few studies I found evaluating women with a combination of stress and urgency incontinence show that Kegels are not as effective for reducing leakage in this population as they are for women with stress incontinence alone.[60] The previously mentioned systematic review found that physical therapy cured symptoms in 35% of women and improved symptoms in 67% of women when any type of urinary incontinence was included in the analysis.[56]

Why don't Kegels improve symptoms for all women, even if they only have stress urinary incontinence? It likely comes down to the extent of muscle damage sustained during childbirth. Unfortunately, it is not standard practice to assess muscle damage using MRI or ultrasound imaging prior to physical therapy treatment. Those types of imaging can reveal whether the levator ani muscles have torn off their anchor points. You cannot increase the strength of a severely torn muscle.

As reported in *BBC Future*, Janis Miller, Professor of Obstetrics and Gynecology at the University of Michigan, said "In the extreme, we're asking for some women to strengthen a muscle they might not even have anymore. What is often observed as pelvic floor weakness is actually a torn muscle."[61]

Since the 1980s, Kegels have become a first line treatment option for women with pelvic organ prolapse as well. Published reviews on the subject state that pelvic floor physical therapy can improve the symptoms and severity of prolapse, among other disorders.[62,63]

Why might Kegels alleviate some symptoms of prolapse? Physical therapists like to use an analogy of a boat in a harbor.[64] The boat *(your uterus, bladder, and rectum)* is held in place by ropes *(ligaments)* tied between the boat and the dock *(your pelvic side walls and sacrum)* and lifted by the water *(your pelvic floor)*. Surely strengthening the "water" would help, right?

Perhaps, if you only have stage I prolapse. If you have stage II prolapse or higher, the boat has already sunk.

In women with fully functioning levator ani muscles, a Kegel squeezes the muscles around the urogenital hiatus shut and provides a lifting force to support her pelvic organs in addition to tightening the external urethral sphincter to stop urine flow. That is why doing 'the Knack,' where you contract and lift your levator ani muscles before coughing, lifting, or landing from a jump can prevent urine leakage. Uninjured young women do not really need to think about this at all though, because that is what their pelvic floor muscles have been reflexively doing for them their whole lives.

In women with severely damaged levator ani muscles and a gaping vagina, the strongest Kegel she can muster will be insufficient to close the urogenital hiatus. Even if she is lying down, with her bottom raised on pillows so that her bulge and cervix are inside her vagina, a Kegel will not close the gap. This is through no fault of her own. It is not due to lack of commitment or doing Kegels wrong. Her muscles are too far gone to be fixed with strength training. Recall what DeLancey wrote, that a 50% or greater loss of levator ani muscle fibers results in disability.

When standing, women with stage II, III, or IV prolapse have an even bigger challenge. Her bulge or cervix is pushing on or protruding beyond the vaginal opening. No Kegel could close the urogenital gap in this scenario. Any increase in intra-abdominal pressure is released through the gap and makes the bulging tissues protrude farther down and out, pulling the uterus down with them.

What pelvic floor physical therapy can potentially do for women with prolapse is reduce painful muscular spasms and improve their sex lives. For some women with prolapse, physical therapy improves their symptoms enough that they don't feel surgery is needed. That is wonderful and makes Kegels worth doing.

I want to make it clear, however, that although worthwhile, Kegels cannot reverse pelvic organ prolapse. I have received a lot of conflicting information on this point, so here is the truth for you. Prolapse is a hernia. Kegels cannot fix the hernia. The only thing that can fix it is surgery.

What I would love to see are more studies aimed at predicting who will benefit from the standard of physical therapy care – Kegel exercises – and who needs something more. These findings could be used to provide individualized care. Perhaps it is unreasonable to have every woman with a pelvic floor disorder sent for an MRI scan. If unjustifiable cost or use of valuable resources is a concern, perhaps only those women who do not see improvement of symptoms after pelvic floor muscle training could be referred for imaging as a next step.

I would also like to see more physical therapists rigorously testing innovative approaches. There are new additions to physical therapy, such as biofeedback and nerve stimulation, but these innovations are always centered around Kegels. Why are we still optimizing the same approach that was first documented in 1948? I am not sure why pelvic floor muscle training is focused only on the levator ani muscles, which are often damaged in women presenting with pelvic floor disorder symptoms, when the levator ani muscles are part of a larger support system.

Looking to human movement science and sports medicine for inspiration, I see that the levator ani muscles are part of the Intrinsic Core, also called the Intrinsic Stabilization System.

The Intrisic Core is the internal cylinder formed by the muscular diaphragm below your lungs, the transverse abdominis muscles along your abdomen, the pelvic floor levator ani muscles and coccygeal muscles, and the multifidus muscle along your spine. Interestingly, the fascia associated with these muscles is connected, creating a sealed core. For example, the abdominal fascia is continuous with investing fascia of diaphragm and pelvic floor. This integrated system of four muscles and their associated fascia enables us to increase intra-abdominal pressure. It is why taking a deep belly breath relaxes and expands your pelvic floor, while exhaling fully contracts the pelvic floor.

When this system is compromised, such as when the pelvic floor muscles are torn or pelvic organ prolapse opens the core to external air pressure, we are no longer able to generate sufficient intra-abdominal pressure to adequately void our bladder or bowels. This causes urine retention and constipation.

For women who have been living for years or decades with a torn pelvic floor, it is certain that the other muscles of the Intrinsic Core have been working double time to compensate. This may in turn affect other systems that the Intrinsic Core interacts with. According to the Brookbush Institute, inhibition of the Intrinsic Core most often results in an increase in synergistic muscle activity of the Anterior Oblique Subsystem, which includes the internal oblique, external oblique, adductor complex, and hip external rotators.[65] I encourage pelvic floor physical therapists to start thinking about how our levator ani muscles fit into these larger systems, and how that knowledge can be used to improve pelvic floor disorder treatments. Perhaps something as simple as a daily deep-breathing practice would strengthen the Intrinsic Core and improve symptoms.

It looks like some physical therapists are starting to publish research on these ideas.[66] There is one interesting study showing that flexing and pointing your toes, especially while standing, activates the pelvic floor muscles, and that core muscles coactivate with pelvic floor muscles.[67]

Hypopressive breathing, also called abdominal vacuum, has been of interest for pelvic floor physical therapy since it contracts the deep core muscles and contracts and lifts the pelvic floor muscles and supportive fascia. To try it, exhale completely and use your core muscles to contract your abdomen to its smallest possible volume. It should feel like your belly button is pushing toward your spine. While holding your core in this contraction, inhale and expand your rib cage. You should feel your stomach suck in even further and your pelvic diaphragm lift as you inhale. This technique can be done lying down, sitting, standing, during forward fold, and more. Though hypopressive exercises are thought to be less effective for pelvic floor strengthening than targeted strengthening with Kegels, it may be a helpful alternative for women whose levator ani muscles are severely damaged, or a beneficial addition to Kegels for all women looking to increase core strength and stability.[69–71]

I am just going to throw another idea out there. It may be that muscle strength is not the only thing that matters for reduction of pelvic floor disorder symptoms. Perhaps a better measure is muscle endurance. Or maybe the angle of muscle action affects the outcome. Would adding a forward or backward pelvic tilt improve the efficacy of Kegels in some women? Keep an open mind. What other factors might contribute to good outcomes? Is there any way to measure them?

It may be that physical therapists with an independent practice are already using this knowledge to improve core stability and to provide women with techniques to increase intra-abdominal pressure during urination and bowel movements. Through large medical institution insurance-provided care, I never once have heard any other muscles beyond the pelvic floor mentioned, or any exercises suggested beyond Kegels.

I would also like to see more studies aimed at understanding whether pelvic floor exercises are protective. The data so far shows that Kegel training during the prenatal period does not prevent *(or cause)* damage from vaginal delivery, but may help those with stress urinary incontinence to reduce symptoms during and after pregnancy.[72,73]

Perhaps Kegels would be protective for women who get C-sections, but to my knowledge this is not known. Carrying a baby is enough strain on the pelvic floor to cause pelvic floor disorders even if vaginal delivery is avoided, but perhaps prenatal Kegels would prevent this. One intriguing study found that prenatal training in Sophrology childbirth *(breathing exercises, body awareness, mindfulness, and meditation)*, Kegel exercises, and Lamaze respiratory training improved maternal health by promoting postpartum pelvic floor function, reducing the incidence of depression, and enhancing sexual function.[74]

How about aging? Can a daily physical therapy regimen prevent the development of symptomatic pelvic floor disorders in aging women? I have not found a satisfactory answer to this question.

For women with fecal incontinence, Kegel exercises can increase the strength of the puborectalis band of the levator ani, assuming it was not damaged too badly. Recall that this band of the levator ani forms a sling around the rectum and is important for continence *(see Chapter 1 and Appendix A)*. However, for most women with fecal incontinence Kegels alone will not fix the problem, because one or both of their sphincters were torn during childbirth.

Physical therapy with biofeedback can reduce fecal incontinence for some women. Biofeedback is helpful in learning how it feels to contract your external sphincter. You can then do contraction repetitions to increase strength. This therapy works best for women who have some sensation of an impending bowel movement. That way you can feel the bowel movement coming and contract your external sphincter until you make it to the toilet.

Sacral nerve stimulation can be a beneficial addition to physical therapy for both urinary and fecal incontinence, especially for women experiencing urgency. Sacral nerves of the pelvis exit the spinal cord at the S3 nerve root of the sacrum and innervate the internal and external anal sphincters, rectum, anal canal, and pelvic floor. They have sensory and motor functions that control the release of feces. For unknown reasons, chronic stimulation of the sacral nerves improves nervous system control of bowel movements.

After a test period to see if your symptoms improve with minimally invasive sacral nerve stimulation, you may be approved for surgical implantation of a sacral nerve stimulation device. The device controls and powers an electrode that delivers electrical pulses to the sacral nerves. Sacral nerve stimulation has been called a "pacemaker for the bladder and bowels." It sounds wild, but it is effective, and it is a needed option for women who fail to remedy their fecal incontinence in other ways.[75-77]

Still complaining of the same problems nearly two years after my daughter was born, I visited my favorite person at the obstetrics and gynecology office, a nurse practitioner. She listened to my concerns and referred me to a physical therapist.

My physical therapist had me lie on my back with knees bent and inserted a lubed, gloved finger into my vagina. Then she asked me to do a Kegel. I did one. She gave me advice on how to do a better one. "Imagine that your vagina is an elevator," she said. "As you do your Kegel, imagine that you are closing the doors to the elevator and lifting it up." I did it again. Then she taught me a simple set of exercises, all a variety on the Kegel, that I could do every day to strengthen my pelvic floor muscles.

Specifically, she told me to lie down, elevate my hips with pillows, and do a set of 10 "long-hold" Kegels, lifting up and in, holding for 5 seconds, then making sure to relax completely before doing another one. Then I was to do a set of 5 "quick flick" Kegels, quickly contracting and releasing. Five years later I saw a different physical therapist who gave me this same therapy plan.

Once you have mastered doing Kegels as above, you can increase the number of repetitions and try them while sitting and standing in addition to on your back. You can also work on getting in the Knack habit. Whenever you feel a cough coming on, do a Kegel and keep your pelvic floor contracted during the cough. Whenever you need to lift something, do a Kegel, and keep your pelvic floor contracted as you lift.

I did these exercises. They did not improve my urinary incontinence or the severity of my prolapse. I found the Knack humorous. When your bladder is at or below your vaginal opening, a Kegel is more likely to squeeze some urine out than to prevent its exit. It was not a waste of effort, though. Kegels did increase the strength of my remaining pelvic muscles enough to improve my sex life.

Pelvic floor exercises improve symptoms for many women and are therefore worth a try. It was worth a try for me, as I intended to have a second baby and was not ready to think about surgery. However, the experience could be improved by setting reasonable expectations and making Kegels enjoyable.

I would have appreciated hearing my gynecologists and physical therapists tell me that pelvic floor exercises have been shown to improve symptoms for some women and are therefore worth a try. I would have been encouraged to commit to doing my daily Kegel exercises if asked to do so for a trial period, after which I would be assessed to see if I am one of the women who will benefit from pelvic floor strengthening or not. Ideally, I would have liked my doctors to follow these steps:

1. Assess my muscle strength with an intravaginal device that senses the electrical activity of muscle contractions *(electromyography, or EMG)*.

2. Train me to do pelvic floor exercises with the intravaginal device in place so I get visual feedback about what is working.

3. Tell me to do these exercises every day without fail for two weeks. Why two weeks? Short enough to commit to and to

feel the pressure of doing it every day, long enough to see results.

4. Have me return to reassess my muscle strength and symptoms to see if there is any improvement. If there is, great! Create a long-term physical therapy plan. If there is not, image my pelvic floor to assess my tissue damage. Talk to me about other therapies I can try. Suggest behavior changes that can make me more comfortable and improve my quality of life until I am ready to consider surgery.

Now, about making Kegels an enjoyable, integrated part of your daily life. I believe that inserting something into the vagina is critical to the success of pelvic floor exercises, and so did Arnold Kegel. He invented the first device that measured Kegel strength, a perineometer.

Want to know if your own Kegels are working? Stick your finger into your vagina and see if you can feel the muscles that surround your vaginal opening contracting and pulling inward. Want to track your increased strength? Stick a device in there that can measure your muscle contractions. There are a number of Bluetooth-enabled Kegel trainers available for purchase now.[78] Simply insert the device into your vagina and Kegel away. The device measures your pelvic floor strength and sends the data to a gamified app in your smartphone.

Bottom line, a finger, measuring device, or dildo gives you something to pull your muscles tightly around, providing valuable feedback. Feeling and seeing your strength increase over time can be hugely motivating.

If you have prolapse, inserting something into your vagina is even more important, because it can push your organs into place while you do your Kegels. That way you strengthen the muscles around a more desirable configuration of body parts. You can also lie down and place pillows under your butt so that your organs fall inward.

Want to have a really good time while doing Kegels? Stick a dildo in there and Kegel your way to orgasm *(simultaneous clito-*

ral stimulation likely needed). Then do more Kegels after you orgasm, while you have increased blood flow and sensation in the
area. Personally, I prefer a hand-blown glass dildo, because it is a
heavy and non-reactive material, and they look like works of art.

Aside from helping with pelvic floor disorders, Kegels can
improve sexual function and increase pleasure. What is per-
ceived as vaginal tightness is actually the pelvic floor muscles
contracting around the penis or other object being inserted
into the vagina. Repetitively gripping an inserted object with
your pelvic floor increases blood flow and the amount of pleasure you feel. Remember the "vaginal sphincter" AKA the bulbospongiosus? It is one of two muscles that loop around your
urethra and vagina in an effort to keep your urogenital hiatus
shut. It also interacts with your clitoris, making it swell when
you are aroused, and contracts at a rapid rate during orgasm. I
couldn't close my urogenital hiatus, but I could definitely still
grip around a dildo.

If sexualizing your Kegels does not sound fun to you, another option is to incorporate them into your daily exercise. Kegels
pair well with certain yoga positions, such as downward dog,
cat/cow, goddess pose, garland pose, child's pose, and legs up
the wall *(the easiest being those last two).* Focus on your breathing and do a Kegel with each exhale. Inhale deeply, relaxing and
expanding your pelvic floor, then exhale, contracting and lifting
the pelvic floor while drawing in the abs slightly.

If you prefer a different kind of exercise, add some stretching at the end and do your Kegels while you stretch. I like to do
them with a seated hamstring stretch or butterfly stretch, or any
of the previously mentioned yoga poses.

If these options do not work for you, think about something
you already do every day that would pair well with Kegels. For
example, you can get in the habit of doing Kegels while you are
in the bath or shower. Bath Kegels with prolapse are interesting,
because you can feel the water entering your vagina and flowing
back out as you expand and contract the pelvic diaphragm.

Another option is to get in the habit of doing Kegels when-ever you are waiting for something, whether that is waiting in line, waiting for your bus stop, waiting for your child to fall asleep, waiting for your toothbrush timer to tell you that your three minutes are up, or waiting for a commercial to end. You get the picture. The goal is to make Kegels a daily habit by inte-grating them with an existing daily habit. That way you do not have to create an additional block of time just for doing Kegels.

To summarize, commit to giving Kegels a try. Do your exer-cises every day for a few weeks and track your symptoms to see if they get any better. Complete the PFDI-20 questionnaire in Appendix D before and after your training. Write down your incontinence symptoms on day 0, 7, and 14. Did any urine leak out today? If yes, what caused it? How much volume came out? Did you have to wear incontinence pads? How many times did you need to change the pad? Did you ever get your underwear or pants wet? How would you rate your libido and ability to orgasm on a scale of 0-4?

You can track your muscle strength by visiting a physical therapist before and after your trial period. This is not necessary, as you will have a sense of whether you are getting stronger or not without a measurement, but can be motivating. Make sure to ask that they measure your muscle strength with an intravag-inal EMG device. You may even want to check in before your appointment to let them know you want to get measurements, just to make sure that is something they can do, and that they will have a device available for you on the day of your visit. Al-ternatively, you can purchase your own Bluetooth Kegel trainer, which are typically a few hundred dollars.

For women who only suffer from stress incontinence, the most common pelvic floor disorder, the majority of those who commit to Kegel training will lessen or cure their leakage prob-lem. For women with multiple types of urinary incontinence, fecal incontinence, or prolapse, give Kegels a try. You may be among the lucky ones whose symptoms improve. Kegels will not fix the source of your problems, but they might just improve the quality of your life.

CHAPTER 6

"PROLAPSE IS A HERNIA"

The two years between my physical therapy attempt and my decision to have a second baby was a period I like to call acceptance light. I accepted that I couldn't do anything to change my body and so I needed to learn to live that way with as little physical and mental distress as possible. I never succeeded completely, but at least I didn't have false hope anymore.

I had two prolapse related concerns about getting pregnant with baby two. First, how would I get sperm inside my uterus when my cervix is hanging outside my body? Second, how the heck was I going to carry this baby with my uterus so low?

The first was an easy fix. I simply used gravity to my advantage. Immediately after sex I would elevate my butt by placing several pillows underneath and lie like that for about twenty minutes. In this position my uterus would fall further into my body, leaving my cervix in the sperm pool long enough that some might make it inside. It took a while, maybe six months, but I got pregnant.

My second concern about carrying the weight of a developing fetus with prolapse really scared me. I was worried about the physical strain and scared for the safety of the fetus. I googled it, of course, and read a few comforting stories on message boards.

I was further comforted by my new gynecologist. I had moved and was lucky to be placed with an excellent gynecologist who was knowledgeable about pelvic floor disorders. I discussed my concern with her, and she told me not to worry.

Even so, that first trimester was rough. My cervix remained low and sunk even lower during those twelve weeks. It seemed unsafe, like foreign agents might invade the protected space. The weight on my bladder and vulva was intense, and my vestibulodynia flared up big time. Then my uterus started to lift. By twenty weeks my baby was tucked up safely inside of me and I had something I had missed dearly — vagina while standing. The remainder of my pregnancy was incredible. I felt better than I had in years.

I carried my second child to 40 weeks with no problems. I again opted for an unmedicated labor and delivery in a hospital setting. I stood and knelt more this time, to encourage his movement downward. When I felt him drop down, I told them I was ready, and positioned myself how I wanted on the bed. I was then admonished by the nurse, who said, "Push! Why aren't you pushing? Did you forget how to push?" I didn't need to push. I just took deep breaths and let my body do its job. I got what was promised. This one fell right out.

I was out of bed walking around and eating within an hour of giving birth. I felt empowered and strong.

After I healed from the birth of my son, I found myself at a new low. My bulge protruded slightly out of my gaping vagina. Worse, I now had the problem I had been dreading. I could no longer poop normally.

I knew of the potential for this problem because at my first physical therapist appointment I answered a long questionnaire. On it I saw the question, "Do you have to insert a finger into your vagina or rectum to help empty your bowels?" I remember thinking, 'Holy shit, that sounds terrible. I am so glad that most of my prolapse problems are with my bladder.' Well, my time had come.

I started to notice that some amount of poop was getting stuck in my rectum. It would sit there and dehydrate into a little poop pebble until I physically removed it. First, I would try sticking my finger into my vagina, locating the poop pebble from the other side, and sliding it down and out. If that didn't work, my only option was to stick my finger into my rectum and fish around for the pebble, then pull it out. Yes, this is gross. And unsexy. And very depressing.

I also started having a new problem with my bladder. I wouldn't feel like I needed to pee at all, but upon moving from a seated to standing position urine would flood out without warning.

The worst case of this happened at an airport while I was traveling alone with my two kids. Just after we got through security, I put my shoes on and stood. Pee started flowing. I sat back down. I did a Kegel and stood again. Pee. My thin pee pad was not going to be able to handle this and I didn't have any change of clothes with me. I sat back down. I decided to take one of my son's diapers and stuff it down into my underwear, right there, in full view of all the people going through security. Then I got up and let the urine flow as I walked my kids into the bathroom to get cleaned up.

At my six-week postpartum check-up I told my gynecologist what was happening. She gave me the best explanation to date of exactly what pelvic organ prolapse is, using rolled up paper as a prop to explain the vagina in relation to the other organs and the types of tissue between them that normally keep them separate. She said physical therapy would not fix it, as that in-between tissue was destroyed. "Prolapse is a hernia," she said. "If you came in here with an intestinal hernia, I wouldn't tell you to go home and do a bunch of sit ups. The only way to repair it is with surgery."

She is one of the heroes in my story, because she was the first to adequately explain prolapse to me, and to help me understand that it was not my fault that my prolapse wasn't getting better. I was not doing Kegels wrong or too infrequently. They had no potential to fix my problems in the first place.

We discussed my issues with urine flooding out when moving from a seated to standing position, and I had a long overdue a-ha moment. She taught me the idea of pooling. When your bladder and rectum extend in and down toward the vaginal opening, what you get are pockets *(see Appendix B)*. Urine and feces tend to get stuck, or pool, in these pockets. When urine pools in your bladder pocket it gets stuck until you make certain movements, such as moving from a seated to standing position. Then it spills out. When feces pools in a rectal pocket it gets stuck, dries out, and compacts, turning into a hard stool. This was the cause of my poop pebbles.

I was already in the habit of leaning forward while urinating to compress my bladder, pushing the urine out like a bellows. But now that was not enough. I was retaining so much urine in my bladder pocket that it would spill out without warning. I got in a new habit of reaching a hand around and gently pushing upward on my perineum and bladder bulge while tilting forward a bit. This caused much of the pooled urine to spill out, greatly reducing my leakage problem.

My gynecologist told me that prolapse is common, and that one-third of women have prolapse. I later verified that this is true, or an underestimate if anything. However, most women who have prolapse in their lifetime do not become symptomatic until decades after vaginal delivery. A much smaller percentage of women report having symptomatic prolapse shortly after vaginal delivery.

In a study of prevalence in the United States, symptomatic prolapse was defined as a positive response to the question, "Do you experience bulging or something falling out you can see or feel in the vaginal area?" The percent of women reporting symptomatic pelvic organ prolapse increased from 2.5% after one delivery to 3.7% after two deliveries.[4]

Though the most damage is caused by your first delivery, it is typical for the number and severity of your pelvic floor disorders to increase with subsequent deliveries. The percent of women reporting at least one pelvic floor disorder *(urinary or fecal incontinence, and/or prolapse)* increased from 18.4% after one delivery to 24.6% after two deliveries to 32.4% after three deliveries.

Next, my gynecologist attempted to fit me with a pessary. A pessary is a soft silicone plug that can be inserted into the vagina to push the organs back into place. They come in a variety of shapes so that you can be matched with your best fit. For some women, a pessary can significantly reduce the symptoms of prolapse.

My doctor shared the curious historical fact that Ancient Egyptians used pessaries. Women were likely creating their own pessaries before this time, but Egyptians kept track of their medical knowledge on papyrus scrolls so it is part of the written record. DeLancey wrote, "Women's suffering from pelvic organ prolapse and incontinence have been recorded since the earliest medical writings. Clear descriptions of prolapse are found in the Kahun papyrus *(1835 B.C.E.)*. 'Of a women whose posterior belly and branching of her thighs are painful, say thou it is the falling of the womb.' *(Kahun papyrus, Column 1, Griffiths translation)*." [1]

The Egyptian use of pessaries is mentioned in many reviews of medical history, but I have been unable to find any direct quotes from the source where a pessary was used to hold up prolapsed organs. [79] Instead, pessaries were used to introduce substances into the vagina, more like a suppository than a modern-day pessary. Ancient Egyptian pessaries were used for the purpose of inducing labor, healing the genitals after difficult labor, or preventing unwanted pregnancy. For example, the Kahun papyrus describes the use of pessaries dipped in spermicidal natural substances like acacia gum to prevent unwanted pregnancy, and the Ebers Papyrus describes the use of healing oil for use after delivery as described in the following excerpt. [80]

"Instructions for a lady suffering in her pubic region, her vagina and the region of her vagina which is between her buttocks.

You shall say concerning her: Very swollen due to giving birth.

You should then prepare for her: oil to be soaked into her vagina."

In 400 B.C.E. the prevailing consensus was that the uterus was an independent animal. It was believed that a prolapsed uterus could be convinced to retreat into the vagina through fumigation or pushed into place with half a pomegranate. In 200 A.D., Soranus, recognizing the problems a pomegranate may cause, suggested a thick woolen tampon wrapped in linen and dipped in vinegar be used to push the uterus into place instead.

The first accurate description of female pelvic anatomy was not published until 1543. As a result of this and other medical advancements, pessaries took off as a treatment for prolapse by the end of the 1500s. First were oval shaped pessaries of brass and waxed cork. Then a variety of shapes made of silver and gold. In the 1860s pessaries of even more shapes and sizes were made of vulcanized rubber, thought to be an improvement because of their flexibility.[81] Since the 1900s, surgery has replaced pessaries as the predominant method of treating prolapse, but pessaries are still an option for women who can't or don't want to have surgery. Today pessaries are made of silicone, which is flexible and thought to be safe for intravaginal use. A properly fitted pessary should be comfortable.

Using a pessary was one part of women's collective experience I was unable to share. My doctor tried wedging several types and sizes in there, but the force of my organs pushed each of them right back out. For a pessary to work they need to stay in place during all your usual daily movements. Some types can even be worn during intercourse. Mine came back out even though I was reclining and relaxed. I didn't even make it to sitting up. My doctor told me I had an unfortunate combination

— a short, gaping vagina and a long, hard cervix. I had a feeling that might be the case, given how my body forcefully expelled tampons, but it was still depressing.

I left this appointment devastated. I barely made it to the privacy of my car before I started to cry. It made me sad to hear that harsh but medically accurate description of my genitals. It was hard to be told that my problems were so severe that surgery was my only option. Mostly, though, I was angry. I was angry at my body, and angry at all the doctors I had talked to before this one who were unable to provide me with accurate information.

After that appointment, every time I went to the bathroom or tried to have sex, I thought about how much I hated my body. I was actively angry about it. I got in the habit of saying, "Fuck you, body," to myself when it gave me problems.

This was starting to feel unlivable, and my understanding is that once you have prolapse, things slowly but surely get worse with time.

CHAPTER 7

"THE STRONGEST MOM IN THE WORLD"

About a year after my son was born, I tried exercising again. Out of everything I tried, yoga gave me the most relief. I started practicing Ashtanga yoga and stuck with it this time. Ashtanga is focused on precise poses and controlled movements between them, timed with steady deep breathing. After a few months the vaginal flatus was easier to control, giving me more freedom to do yoga when and where I wished. I could feel that Ashtanga strengthened my pelvic floor more than Kegels alone.

Once I felt strong enough, I started exploring other types of exercise and found aerial silks. Aerial silks is a circus art where a long piece of low-stretch fabric is tied at the middle to a swivel anchor on the ceiling, such that two separate pieces of fabric hang from ceiling to floor. You learn to climb up the silks, wrap yourself in them, and do a variety of poses and tricks. I felt like I had finally found a sport worth doing. I was having so much fun and was soon in the best shape of my life. I felt like I was leveling up in what my body could do.

To any outside observer, I looked strong. My daughter was impressed with my muscles and abilities, telling me regularly that I was the strongest mom in the world. Meanwhile, I was in a private battle with the symptoms of my pelvic floor disorders.

My new sport came with a cost. Inversions, where you use your arm and core strength to flip upside down, are a basic move in aerial silks. These movements seemed to make my prolapse worse than ever. High volumes of urine leakage and poop pebbles became a daily discomfort.

I went back to my gynecologist. She told me that I should not do aerial silks anymore. Her words were an echo of advice I had heard before. I had been advised by multiple doctors and physical therapists that low impact exercise, like swimming or walking, is best for women with pelvic floor disorders.

Having my doctors tell me this created fear that exercise could further damage my body and make my pelvic floor disorders permanently worse. I had the same experience multiple times. I would start to exercise, get worsening symptoms, and stop out of fear. A lot of women express fear of engaging in exercise or even playing with and picking up their children out of fear of worsening symptoms.[46]

Should we be afraid or not? What kinds of exercises can increase the severity of pelvic floor disorders? And if I did get surgery, could these same exercises cause my disorders to return?

For women who have never had children, high impact exercises like long-distance running and gymnastics can cause urinary incontinence during exercise, but this is not lasting. Olympic gymnasts and track and field athletes who had urinary incontinence during their sports careers were not more likely to have incontinence later in life. High impact exercises did not increase the likelihood of having fecal incontinence, with a few exceptions. Being a competitive cheerleader or paratrooper can cause the development of lasting fecal incontinence or prolapse.[82,83] Weight lifting did not affect the likelihood of having any of the three pelvic floor disorders. This suggests that the greatest harm to pelvic floor tissues during exercise is caused by high force of impact during hard landings. Irreparable damage to pelvic floor muscles and connective tissue are likely to blame.

For women who have had children, you can expect that some exercises will cause urine leakage. One study of mothers with urinary incontinence found that certain CrossFit exercises caused urine leakage. Mothers were likely to leak during box jumps, jumping rope *(especially double-unders)*, thrusters, squats without weights, squats with weights, and trampoline jumping. The women in the study had devised simple strategies to avoid embarrassing moments. For example, emptying their bladder before exercising, wearing dark pants, and doing Kegels for extra support during exercises that caused urine leakage.[84]

This study shows that two types of exercise cause leakage — exercises that require a large increase in intra-abdominal pressure *(lifting)* and exercises with a forceful impact of your feet on the floor *(jumping)*. Similar studies have shown that high impact activities such as jumping or running cause the most problems with urine leakage [see [85] for review].

The reason for this has been anatomically studied. With each impact, the bladder neck and genital organs descend. A higher impact causes more descent of the bladder neck, such that it is more likely for urine to leak out.[86]

There are few studies on exercising with symptomatic pelvic organ prolapse or fecal incontinence. The authors of a 2020 review in Sports Medicine wrote, "There is some evidence that strenuous exercise may cause and worsen pelvic organ prolapse, but data are inconsistent."[87] One reason for limited and inconsistent studies seems to be that the technologies to measure intra-abdominal pressure, pelvic floor muscle strength, and the movement of muscles and organs during exercise are still in development. There is no gold standard approach for the small number of researchers asking these questions.

I found just one study that quantified subjective and objective measurements of prolapse after an hour of moderate physical activity.[88] The authors found that 54% of women with prolapse reported a subjective increase in prolapse symptoms and that 26% of them had an objective increase in POP-Q stage after activity. However, there was no clear correlation between these findings. In other words, the women experiencing increased symptoms were not necessarily the same women who had a measurable increase in POP-Q stage. The authors did not determine how long the increase in symptoms lasted.

Since this study looked at moderate activity such as walking, moving from seated to standing, and bending over, it can be assumed that intense activities like running or weight-lifting would cause an increase in prolapse symptoms greater than or equal to that of moderate activity. Increased prolapse and discomfort caused by physical activity are likely temporary, but I can't write that with certainty because it has not been studied.

In summary, if you have a pelvic floor disorder, you can expect that high impact exercises and exercises that increase your intra-abdominal pressure will make the symptoms of your disorder worse, at least during exercise. Whether these effects can be lasting is unclear.

My interpretation of the available data is that exercising with pelvic floor disorders causes discomfort and an exacerbation of symptoms, but that these effects are temporary. Pelvic floor disorders do get worse over time, but the data points to factors other than exercise as the cause. Having more children, gaining a significant amount of weight, and aging will all likely increase the severity of your pelvic floor disorders. Overweight women with pelvic floor disorders who lose a significant amount of weight typically report that their symptoms have decreased. That leaves vaginal birth trauma, aging, and impact related pelvic floor trauma as the only causes of pelvic floor disorders with evidence for permanent effects.

My take? Though uncomfortable and potentially embarrassing, exercise is unlikely to have permanent effects. The forces created by most types of exercise *(hard-impact sports aside)* are nothing compared to vaginal delivery. Just don't take up competitive cheerleading or dirt bike jumping, ok?

Hopefully by the time I write a second edition of this book there will be enough evidence to conclusively back up my claim that there is nothing to fear. Most types of exercise cannot permanently damage your tissues.

Every individual needs to do her own cost-benefit analysis. Do the health benefits of exercise outweigh the cost of increased symptoms during exercise? If your answer is yes, I have some tips for getting back into exercises you haven't done for a while or starting new ones.

If you can't stay away from running, try strengthening your pelvic floor, butt, and core first, either with yoga or a combination of strengthening exercises you enjoy, then gradually introduce running. Start with short distances and increase bit by bit. Avoid concrete and asphalt if you can, as your foot fall on those surfaces create the harshest impact. Try running on dirt or around a track. Your pelvic floor will thank you.

For abdominal exercises, a physical therapist told me that getting in the habit of exhaling as you increase intra-abdominal pressure can help. For example, exhale as you curl up into a crunch, inhale as you lower yourself back to the floor. That way the pressure is released to some extent by your diaphragm moving upward and making more space in the abdominal cavity. Slow, controlled abdominal exercises are better than rapid, high-intensity reps.

It is important to have body awareness as you exercise. Do you find yourself straining during a given exercise? Does your straining cause your organs to descend or your bladder or bowels to leak? If yes, think of how you can modify that exercise to strain less. Do the modified version until you are strong enough to do the full version. Go slow. Start with a low number of reps or light weight and build up slowly.

Women with prolapse cannot count on their levator ani muscles to cushion and lift their organs, since their organs are protruding below the plane of muscle action. Keeping your legs together provides some support. For this reason, squats or splits are especially hard on prolapse.

For any type of exercise, a slow and steady build of difficulty, intensity, and duration is best. Try not to exert yourself in
ways your body is not prepared for. Instead, work up to it slowly.
Consistency is also important. If you go a few weeks or more
without exercising, you will need to be patient and do the slow
and steady build again.

After learning more about exercise and the pelvic floor, here
is how I interpret my experience with aerial silks. During exercise I had an increase in urinary incontinence and prolapse
bulge. Over the following day or so I had a resulting increase
in pooled feces. I also had frequent flare ups of vestibulodynia,
likely caused by wearing tight leggings. These temporary dis-
comforts caused fear that I was further breaking my body.

I wish that I had stuck with the exercises that made me happy and healthy. I did succeed in sticking with yoga, and there
was a period of about six months where I stuck with running. In
both cases, my symptoms initially worsened a lot during exercise. The first 2-4 weeks were hard. Once I got stronger and my
body adapted to that level of effort my symptoms didn't fluctu-
ate so much.

Silks was different because I was constantly leveling up in
difficulty. I was straining and bearing down as I learned to do
inversions to compensate for my lack of abdominal strength. A
better approach would be to strengthen my abs first, to start
with conditioning inversions from the floor where I can jump
up to give myself a boost, or to have someone give me an assist
until I became strong enough to do it myself.

It is unclear whether doing high impact, abdominal, or lifting exercises after surgery would generate strain on your pelvic floor that eventually causes your incontinence or prolapse
symptoms to return. My surgeon told me that it is safe to do
whatever exercise I want once healed from surgical repair. Unfortunately, I could not verify his claim with research, because I
could not find a single research paper on this topic.

My biggest question, can I get back to running and aerial
silks after surgery without worrying that my symptoms will re-

turn, remains inconclusively answered. Based on what I have read, I have decided to go for it. I will be smart about it, and not push myself too hard too fast, but I will not restrict myself from doing any of the exercises I enjoy.

CHAPTER 8

"YOU DID GOOD, UTERUS"

It was time for me to decide. Did I want to have another child, or did I want to get surgery to correct my problems? Having another child would mean more damage to my body and putting off surgery for at least two years. After some deliberation I decided I was ready to let go of the idea of a third child. It was time to create something besides babies. It was time to consider surgery.

My gynecologist referred me to a doctor who specializes in the surgical correction of pelvic floor disorders. It turns out my two heroes are connected. My pelvic floor repair surgeon trained my favorite gynecologist for a time. So much of the quality of my treatment depended on proximity to doctors who understand and care about pelvic floor disorders. This time, luck was on my side.

It was at this point that I first met with my urogynecologist as described in Chapter 1. Almost a year went by between our first visit and my surgery. This was in part because it was difficult to schedule, and in part because he discovered that I had a spasm in one of my pelvic floor muscles. Since women with muscle spasms have more difficult and painful recoveries, he sent me back to physical therapy.

The therapy did not successfully rid me of my spasm. I did learn that propping your bottom up on pillows for twenty minutes once or several times a day helps to temporarily alleviate the feelings of discomfort and pressure from prolapse. It is funny, I guess, to finally learn this trick just before it would no longer be needed.

During the weeks leading up to surgery I was an emotional mess. My stress largely centered around the fact that I was electing to remove my uterus. I didn't want to have more children, right? What would this mean for my identity as a woman? What would it feel like to have my uterus missing? I had an appendectomy about a year prior. Is this what aging is — the gradual removal of failing organs until the system itself fails?

On surgery day the pre-op nurses were understaffed, so I was waiting in a small room by myself for a few hours. I thought about how much I love my children and started to cry. Not out of fear or sadness. I was simply overwhelmed by my love for them. I was grateful to have two healthy, happy kids. I put my hand on my abdomen and thought, "You did good, uterus. Thank you."

My surgery was supposed to last four hours and be an outpatient procedure. Most women feel well enough to go home the day of surgery and have one tough week of pain, tiredness, and difficulty with bowel movements before they feel largely better. I was on the unlucky end of the spectrum, because of my muscle spasms and the unexpected additional procedure I needed. I do not want to scare anyone away from surgery with my story. I had a much harder time that most, but even so, if I went back in time knowing what I know now, I would still choose surgery.

After my surgery was complete, I woke to my husband by my side and my surgeon telling him that I had lost a lot of blood. He had identified a major muscular defect during surgery and had to do more repairs than anticipated. He said that the surgery was a success. I remember shaking his hand to thank him. My husband tells me I asked the surgeon and every nurse who came into the room when I would be able to have sex again, which is hilarious, but I don't remember that or much else from my days in the hospital.

My surgery lasted nearly six hours and included six procedures. I spent two nights in the hospital. It was ten days before I could get around without a walker, and four weeks before I could walk a mile. Most people get their catheter out within a few days after surgery. I had mine for two weeks, resulting in a urinary tract infection, then needed to self-catheterize several times a day for two weeks after that because I was still retaining urine. I still had pain, bruising, and swelling at six weeks, so I had to wait a few more weeks to attempt exercise or intercourse.

Those first two weeks of recovery were brutal. I have a new level 10 on my pain scale. During my initial attempts to walk or poop the pain was worse than having my first child. My entire body would go clammy and I would shake, hyperventilate, and nearly faint.

By day four after surgery I still had not been able to poop, so I took a strong laxative. My first bowel movement came that evening as a completely uncontrolled, painful release of diarrhea. My diarrhea continued periodically through the night and into the next day, but I was too weak to clean up after myself. To think I used to lie to my husband about my problem because it wasn't sexy. Now he has removed my adult diaper and wiped diarrhea off my body. I stopped taking laxatives and regained control of my bowels, but every bowel movement felt like a mini-birth experience for the first two weeks.

It was about two weeks into my recovery that I started writing this book and learning more about what surgical repairs had been made.

To correct my stress urinary incontinence, a laparoscopic procedure was used to place a sling made of non-absorbable, sterile surgical mesh under my urethra. Small incisions were made through the skin above my pubic bone, my only visible scars from my many procedures, and the tiny robot hands of the laparoscope were manipulated to place the mesh. This procedure alone only takes fifteen to thirty minutes and has a fast recovery time. It is definitely worth considering if you have stress incontinence that is not cured with physical therapy.

The mesh used for urethral slings is different from the mesh you may have heard scary reports about. For years, peaking in 2013, surgeons implanted large pieces of mesh to fix anterior prolapse. The mesh was supposed to replace torn fascia and hold prolapsed bladders in place. According to a 2019 report from the FDA, mesh used to treat anterior prolapse has resulted in 10,391 reports of serious injury, 806 reports of device malfunctions, and 77 reports of death.[89] In contrast, a urethral sling is a small piece of mesh intended to hold up the bladder neck so that you are less likely to leak. This approach is proven to have good outcomes. If it doesn't work out it is easy enough to remove.

To correct my uterine prolapse, my surgeon removed my uterus and then resuspended my vagina by attaching it to ligaments. Stealing from the earlier 'boat in a harbor' analogy, ligaments are the ropes holding the boat *(my vagina, in this case)* to the dock *(my body walls)*.

I watched a video of Emily C. Von Bargen, Female Pelvic Medicine and Reconstructive Surgery Associate Fellowship Director at Massachusetts General Hospital, performing this procedure on a 74 year old patient to better understand it.[90] Though her patient went through a significant series of procedures and was 74 years old, she had her foley catheter removed two hours after surgery and was discharged from the hospital the same day. This is a good example of a typical outcome. In another surgical video, also published in the *Journal of Medical Insight*, an 87 year old patient who underwent surgical repair of rectal prolapse had the same uncomplicated outcome.[91]

From what I saw in the surgical video, I imagine doing these surgeries is both challenging and surprising. Challenging because visibility is limited. Aside from the placement of the urethral sling, all my procedures were done through the vagina. It is one thing to look at female pelvis anatomy in a diagram, with all parts and tissue types clearly labeled. It is another to look at the wet, bloody viscera of a living human being through a small opening and get your bearings. Pelvic floor repair can also be surprising, because the surgeon is not completely sure what condition the tissues will be in until they can see them. It has the feeling of a treasure hunt.

First comes the hysterectomy. In my case, this included removal of the cervix, uterus, and fallopian tubes. My ovaries were left in place. The surgeon must cut the vagina, ligaments, fascia, and blood vessels away from the uterus before it can be removed. In the video, Von Bargen used a combination of sharp dissection tools and a blood vessel sealing tool that can grasp, cut, and seal tissues simultaneously, reducing blood loss. With these tools she made her way around the uterus, snipping off all the attachments while protecting the bladder and rectum with metal barriers. Once completed, the uterus, about the size of a small pear, was easily lifted out of the body cavity. Von Bargen noted that the cervix of her patient was elongated, typical of women with pelvic organ prolapse. A healthy cervix is usually about 3.5 centimeters. Mine was noted to be 7 centimeters after it was removed.

24% of women in the United States have had a hysterectomy.[4] Surgery is bizarre. How crazy is it that we can elect to remove an organ, have someone open us up and cut it out, and go on with our lives as normal afterward? When you take a step back and think about it, it seems barbaric.

We are better off than women who came before us. The first hysterectomy took place in 1507, and was accomplished by tying rope tightly around the uterus until it became gangrenous and fell out.[79]

Over time surgeons have developed more precise instruments and a better understanding of human anatomy, but the basics of surgery remain the same. Cut out the irreparably broken or unneeded parts. Reconnect the cut or torn parts. For all its crudeness, surgery works remarkably well. Once a surgeon reconnects the severed tissues of the female pelvis the body gets to work and strengthens the repair.

Surgeons have started advancing into the next phase now, creating biocompatible synthetic parts and engineered biological parts to replace our damaged parts. I look forward to the day when these approaches can be combined with molecular tools for tissue regeneration and repair. Perhaps the pessary of the future will deliver a healing mixture of small molecules to the pelvis immediately after childbirth. Perhaps the tissue grafts of the future will be embedded with proteins that encourage tissue healing and strength.

After the removal of my cervix, uterus, and fallopian tubes was complete, my vagina had two open ends: the usual opening to the outside, and a new opening where it used to be attached to the cervix. If the interior opening is simply sutured shut as is, the vagina will not have any structure to hold it up. To solve this problem, surgeons do what they call "uterosacral ligament suspension" to create what I call a "vagina tent."

The uterus is held up by two uterosacral ligaments, which extend from the uterus up to an attachment point on a bone at the base of our spine called the sacrum. During hysterectomy, the ligaments are cut away from the uterus so that the uterus can be removed. To create a vagina tent, these ligaments are re-purposed to suspend the vagina. When the interior end of the vagina is sutured shut, the uterosacral ligaments are sealed into the closure so that they hold the vagina up. Voila, an A-Frame vagina tent.

To correct my prolapsed bladder, the anterior vaginal wall was cut open and dissected away from the pubocervical fascia so that any defects in the fascia — tears or avulsions away from the anchor points — could be identified and sutured shut. Large defects may require a tissue graft. The graft of choice these days is cadaver skin, processed to remove any molecular memory of its source so there is no chance of rejection.

I recall laughing to myself when I first heard this, imagining that I would have a patchwork cadaver-skin vagina, and feeling grateful that my husband and I are both scientists who would not be bothered by such a thing, but my imagination was not accurate. I thought the cadaver skin would be used to patch up the vagina itself, but it was not. The cadaver skin was used to patch up the torn fascia between the vagina and other pelvic organs. So, no worries, your partner's penis will not be rubbing up against a dead person's tissues. Well, not directly contacting them anyway.

During my anterior repair, my surgeon found that I had a tear down the midline of my fascia as well as a paravaginal defect, where the fascia tears away from its anchor points on both sides of the body. A paravaginal defect is a common enough result of childbirth to have a name, and is known to cause anterior prolapse.[92]

The bladder is held up by a hammock of fascia attached along two lines of dense connective tissue called the arcus tendineus (see Appendix A). A hammock that is not attached to sturdy anchor points no longer functions as a hammock, and drops whatever was relying on it for support. In a paravaginal defect, the fascia has ripped off of the arcus tendineus on both sides, dropping the bladder.

A large, 10-centimeter graft of cadaver skin was needed to repair my fascia hammock completely. Once the midline tear was stitched together and the graft was sewn into place, the surgical cut of my vagina was sutured shut.

My surgeon also found that I needed posterior repair for a large rectal prolapse, as predicted. This was achieved by giving me an episiotomy from the perineum to just above the level of my prolapsed rectum. The posterior vaginal wall was dissected away from my rectovaginal fascia so that the tears could be sutured shut.

The irony that I ended up getting an episiotomy after all is not lost on me.

During this part of my surgical treasure hunt, my surgeon found a surprise — a large muscular defect. His surgery notes say simply that I had a "significantly attenuated proximal perineal body," and that "the defect was noted to be very large."

He explained at a follow up appointment. The perineal body, an anchor point for multiple bands of pelvic floor muscles just under the perineum, should be thick with muscle *(see Appendix A)*. In my case there was nothing there but skin. The muscles had completely torn away, likely during the birth of my first child, and were hanging uselessly in the wrong location. He had to surgically reconstruct my perineal body and attach each torn off band of muscle back to it. He said he had not seen a defect that large in a long time.

Let us take a moment to reflect. The delivery of my first child tore the anterior fascia along the midline and away from the anchor points on both sides, tore my posterior fascia along the midline, and tore my pelvic floor muscles away from the perineal body.

Can we say it together now? Kegels are not going to fix this. There was never any chance that they would.

CHAPTER 9

ROOM FOR IMPROVEMENT

Why hadn't I ever heard of pelvic floor disorders before giving birth? Why didn't I know the extent of bodily damage caused by childbirth until over seven years after the fact, even though I spoke to ten different doctors about my symptoms? Something is wrong here.

There is a lot of room for improvement and innovation in women's health. As I wrote in Chapter 2, every pregnant woman should be told that giving birth may result in damage to her pelvic floor tissues. They should be informed about what symptoms to look out for and discuss with their doctor during the postpartum period. All that is needed is a group of doctors who care enough about making this standard protocol to push for institution-wide change.

As I wrote in Chapter 3, couples should be advised that a decrease in sexual activity is to be expected for at least the first year following childbirth. Decreased sex is not due to lack of interest, but to injury. Delivery causes very real damage to pelvic floor muscles, connective tissues, and nerves. Damaged tissues can take a long time to heal and may cause pain and inflammation during or after intercourse for up to a year after childbirth. For most of the 85% of women who tear their perineum during childbirth, the pain should subside within 6 months of delivery. If still experiencing pain beyond 6 months, women should be referred to a urogynecologist who can identify the source of pain during intercourse and come up with an appropriate treatment plan.

During the postpartum period, women should be asked about any pelvic floor disorder symptoms and how they affect their quality of life, either directly or through a survey. Postpartum women should also be asked about depression and substance abuse, and an intervention should be offered if there is evidence of either, as discussed in Chapter 4.

A review as recent as 2018 declared that there isn't even an adequate pelvic floor disorder questionnaire in existence for your obstetrician gynecologist to give you, writing that, "There is no questionnaire that is highly recommended to assess the pelvic floor disorder in a complete and integrated way by the International Consultation on Incontinence." [93] See Appendix D for examples of commonly used questionnaires. They are fine, but no single questionnaire addresses all pelvic floor disorders and their impact on your quality of life. Giving patients such a form should be routine practice at the first postpartum checkup.

When women present with symptoms of pelvic floor disorders, they should be referred to a urogynecologist immediately. The psychological toll and other quality of life effects are too great to delay. In addition to standard urogynecology assessments, perhaps magnetic resonance imaging or ultrasound imaging of pelvic anatomy should be routinely used to assess the amount of structural damage.[94]

As discussed in Chapter 5, since physical therapy does not work for everyone, that should be explained up front. Motivation to commit to a trial period of Kegel exercises would be encouraged by clearly stated physical therapy goals and objective measures of outcomes. Women who don't have any improvement in their symptoms after physical therapy need MRI or ultrasound imaging to assess tissue damage. Ideally this would happen sooner, such as when first referred to a urogynecologist, but better late than never. As Janis Miller said in an interview for *BBC Future*, "Diagnosing birth injuries is key to individualising treatment."[61]

I also want to question something that always puzzled me: why are we assessed for prolapse while lying down? A couple of coughs is not enough. Don't you need to see how gravity affects the displacement of my organs in order to understand the severity of my prolapse?

I have the same question for physical therapy. Why is our pelvic floor strength assessed while we are lying down? And why are we only taught to do a Kegel in this position? Also, a vaginal device to measure muscle strength is a great start, but why are we still optimizing this one idea from 1948? Even the basic measurements of resting pelvic floor muscle tone and strength of contraction are not routinely done in every physical therapy office for every patient. We can do so much better than this.

Why not outfit us with sensors and see what our pelvic floor muscles and organs are doing while sitting and standing, and how they respond to common movements – getting up, sitting down, walking, lifting, jumping, and running. What if you could see what is happening inside of us during physical therapy muscle training? What if you could have many measurable outcomes of a given training period? Wouldn't that information help to optimize therapy for each individual? There are some studies using surface muscle contraction sensors to measure muscle activation.[67,95,96] How about accelerometers? Would those be useful to measure pelvic floor movement and possibly pelvic organ descent?[97]

Looking ahead, we need to move toward a future where measurable risk factors are identified and can be used to predict who is likely develop a severe pelvic floor disorder because of vaginal delivery. The best preventative strategies need to be determined so that women in this situation have options for their care. Pregnant women would be individually assessed for these to-be-determined risk factors and informed of to-be-determined alternative options to vaginal delivery.

Currently, elective C-section seems to be the best option for prevention. We should not be satisfied with this solution, though. C-sections are major surgeries with their own list of risks. What is really needed are innovative treatments for pelvic floor injury that could be administered immediately following childbirth.

So far, there is one peculiar quality thought to put women at greater risk of developing severe pelvic organ prolapse — hypermobility.[98–100] Women who are hypermobile have differences in the structure and function of their connective tissues down to the molecular level.[101] Their fascia and ligaments, the connective tissues that compartmentalize and suspend pelvic organs, are more likely to tear or stretch beyond repair during delivery. Well, add me to that data set, because I am hypermobile, and, wow, did I tear and stretch.

My daughter is more hypermobile than I am, as she inherited this trait from both sides. I am scared for her, but at this time I do not have any clear advice to give her.

If you are training to be a doctor, please consider joining the effort to improve women's health. We need you.

If you are one of my sisters in suffering and want to help improve women's health, consider volunteering your time as a research subject. You can elect to answer surveys, take part in experiments to improve the diagnosis and treatment of pelvic floor disorders, or both. Email me at georgeann@georgeannsack.com with your name and preferred method of contact and I will add you to a list of interested participants.

As my surgeon predicted, now that I have fully recovered the pain I experienced after surgery seems like a long, bad dream. It is too soon to tell whether the surgical fixes will hold for a lifetime, but for now the repairs were successful.

I have no bulge. No protruding cervix. No pressure on my labia causing chronic pain and discomfort. I am no longer embarrassed by the appearance and dysfunction of my genitals. I can pee and poop normally, without using my hand or finger for assistance or worrying that a flood of urine is going to spill out when I stand up. I can run and jump without leaking urine. I don't need to wear pee pads anymore, which means less vulvar irritation and more pretty underwear.

I have functioning pelvic floor muscles. Sex feels good again. So good. I cried the first time it felt so good.

The absence of my uterus is not noticeable during daily activities or intercourse and has not caused any sadness or stress. I am no less of a woman. I feel more proud to be a woman than ever before.

Whatever the future brings, I will enjoy this time. I know my body now. Armed with an understanding of my pelvic health, I am prepared for any outcome.

BIBLIOGRAPHY

1. DeLancey JOL. 2010. "Current status of the subspecialty of female pelvic medicine and reconstructive surgery." *Am J Obstet Gynecol. 202(6)*:658.e1-658.e4.

2. Steers WD. 2013. "Establishing the subspecialty of female pelvic medicine and reconstructive surgery in the United States of America." *Arab J Urol.* 11*(2)*:113-116.

3. DeLancey JOL. 2017. "Mommy, how will the baby get out of your tummy? Will it hurt you?" *Am J Obstet Gynecol. 217(2)*:110-111.

4. Wu JM, Vaughan CP, Goode PS, Redden DT, Burgio KL, Richter HE, Markland AD. 2014. "Prevalence and trends of symptomatic pelvic floor disorders in U.S. women." *Obstet Gynecol.* 123*(1)*:141-148.

5. Dheresa M, Worku A, Oljira L, Mengistie B, Assefa N, Berhane Y. 2020. "Women's health seeking behavior for pelvic floor disorders and its associated factors in eastern Ethiopia." *Int Urogynecol J.* April 2020.

6. Chen CCG, Avondstondt AM, Khatry SK, Singh M, Klasen EM, LeClerq SC, Katz J, Tielsch JM, Mullany LC. 2019. "Prevalence of symptomatic urinary incontinence and pelvic organ prolapse among women in rural Nepal." *Int Urogynecol J.* December 2019.

7. Hakimi S, Aminian E, Mohammadi M, Mohammad Alizadeh S, Bastani P, Houshmandi S. 2020. "Prevalence and risk factors of urinary/anal incontinence and pelvic organ prolapse in healthy middle-aged iranian women." *J Menopausal Med.* 26*(1)*:24.

8. Shen L, Yang J, Bai X, Sun Z. 2020. "Analysis of the current status of pelvic floor dysfunction in urban women in Xi'an City." *Ann Palliat Med.* 9*(5)*:25-25.

9. Geirsson RT. 1986 "Intrauterine volume in pregnancy." *Acta Obstet Gynecol Scand Suppl.* 136:1-74.

10. Gao H, Liu D, Li Y, Tang J, Wu X, Tan H. 2019. "Uterine size and volume are associated with higher live birth rate in patients undergoing assisted reproduction technology." *Medicine (Baltimore).* 98*(47)*:e17966.

11. Centers for Disease Control and Prevention. "Clinical growth charts." https://www.cdc.gov/growthcharts/clinical_charts.htm.

12. Burnett LA, Cook M, Shah S, Michelle Wong M, Kado DM, Alperin M. 2020. "Age-associated changes in the mechanical properties of human cadaveric pelvic floor muscles." *J Biomech.* 98:109436.

13. Reddy RA, Cortessis V, Dancz C, Klutke J, Stanczyk FZ. 2020. "Role of sex steroid hormones in pelvic organ prolapse." *Menopause.* April 2020:1.

14. Manresa M, Pereda A, Bataller E, Terre-Rull C, Ismail KM, Webb SS. 2019. "Incidence of perineal pain and dyspareunia following spontaneous vaginal birth: a systematic review and meta-analysis." *Int Urogynecol J.* 30*(6)*:853-868.

15. DeLancey JOL. 2016. "What's new in the functional anatomy of pelvic organ prolapse?" *Curr Opin Obstet Gynecol.* 28*(5)*:420-429.

16. Samarasekera DN, Bekhit MT, Wright Y, Lowndes RH, Stanley KP, Preston JP, Preston P, Speakman CTM. 2008. "Long-term anal continence and quality of life following postpartum anal sphincter injury." *Color Dis.* 10*(8)*:793-799.

17. Stenson AL. 2017. "Vulvodynia." *Obstet Gynecol Clin North Am.* 44*(3)*:493-508.

18. Butwick AJ, Wong CA, Guo N. 2018. "Maternal body mass index and use of labor neuraxial analgesia." *Anesthesiology.* 129*(3)*:448-458.

19. Health Care Foundation C. 2018. "Listening to mothers in California: Results from a population-based survey of women's childbearing experiences data snapshot 2." *Listening to Mothers in California*. September 2018. www.chcf.org.

20. Gaskin IM. 2003. *Ina May's Guide To Childbirth*. New York: Bantam Books.

21. Chaliha C. 2009. "Postpartum pelvic floor trauma." *Curr Opin Obstet Gynecol*. 21*(6)*:474-479.

22. Smith LA, Price N, Simonite V, Burns EE. 2013. "Incidence of and risk factors for perineal trauma: a prospective observational study." *BMC Pregnancy Childbirth*. 13*(1)*:59.

23. Handa VL. 2019. "Effect of pregnancy and childbirth on urinary incontinence and pelvic organ prolapse." *UpToDate*. Accessed June 2020.

24. Berkowitz L, Foust-Wright C. 2018. "Postpartum perineal care and management of complications." *UpToDate*. Accessed June 2020.

25. Hilde G, Stær-Jensen J, Siafarikas F, Engh ME, Brækken IH, Bo K. 2013. "Impact of childbirth and mode of delivery on vaginal resting pressure and on pelvic floor muscle strength and endurance." *Am J Obstet Gynecol*. 208*(1)*:50.e1-50.e7.

26. Roser M, Ritchie H. "Maternal mortality. Our world in data. https://ourworldindata.org/maternal-mortality. Accessed June 2020.

27. Oster E. 2019. "Why the C-section rate is so high." *The Atlantic*. https://www.theatlantic.com/ideas/archive/2019/10/c-section-rate-high/600172/

28. O'Donnell B. 2008. "We know the reality of childbirth." *The Guardian*. https://www.theguardian.com/society/2008/jul/11/nhs.health1

29. Handa VL, Blomquist JL, Knoepp LR, Hoskey KA, McDermott KC, Muñoz A. 2011. "Pelvic floor disorders 5–10 years after vaginal or Cesarean childbirth." *Obstet Gynecol*. 118*(4)*:777-784.

30. Blomquist JL, Muñoz A, Carroll M, Handa VL. 2018. "Association of delivery mode with pelvic floor disorders after childbirth." *JAMA.* 320*(23)*:2438.

31. Larsson C, Källen K, Andolf E. 2009. "Cesarean section and risk of pelvic organ prolapse: a nested case-control study." *Am J Obstet Gynecol.* 200*(3)*:243.e1-243.e4.

32. WHO. 2015. "WHO statement on caesarean section rates." https://www.who.int/reproductivehealth/publications/maternal_perinatal_health/cs-statement/en/

33. Khajehei M, Doherty M, Tilley PJM, Sauer K. 2015. "Prevalence and risk factors of sexual dysfunction in postpartum Australian women." *J Sex Med.* 12*(6)*:1415-1426.

34. Lagaert L, Weyers S, Van Kerrebroeck H, Elaut E. 2017. "Postpartum dyspareunia and sexual functioning: a prospective cohort study." *Eur J Contracept Reprod Heal Care.* 22*(3)*:200-206.

35. Urbankova I, Grohregin K, Hanacek J, Krcmar M, Feyereisl J, Deprest J, Krofta L. 2019. "The effect of the first vaginal birth on pelvic floor anatomy and dysfunction." *Int Urogynecol J.* 30*(10)*:1689-1696.

36. Anglès-Acedo S, Ros-Cerro C, Escura-Sancho S, Elías-Santo-Domingo N, Palau-Pascual MJ, Espuña-Pons M. 2019. "Coital resumption after delivery among OASIS patients: differences between instrumental and spontaneous delivery." *BMC Womens Health.* 19*(1)*:154.

37. Yeniel AO, Petri E. 2014. "Pregnancy, childbirth, and sexual function: perceptions and facts." *Int Urogynecol J.* 25*(1)*:5-14.

38. Reamy KJ, White SE. 1987. "Sexuality in the puerperium: A review." *Arch Sex Behav.* 16*(2)*:165-186.

39. Barbara G, Pifarotti P, Facchin F, Cortinovis I, Dridi D, Ronchetti C, Calzolari L, Vercellini P. 2016. "Impact of mode of delivery on female postpartum sexual functioning: Spontaneous vaginal delivery and operative vaginal delivery vs Cesarean section." *J Sex Med.* 13*(3)*:393-401.

40. Herman and Wallace. "Orthopedic considerations for sexual activity." https://hermanwallace.com/products/orthopedic-considerations-for-sexual-activity.

41. Centers for Disease Control and Prevention. 2019. "Preventing excessive alcohol consumption." *Alcohol and Public Health.* http://www.thecommunityguide.org/alcohol/index.html.

42. Zhu Q, Shu H, Dai Z. 2019. "Effect of pelvic floor dysfunction on sexual function and quality of life in Chinese women of different ages: An observational study." *Geriatr Gerontol Int.* 19*(4)*:299-304.

43. Mazi B, Kaddour O, Al-Badr A. 2019. "Depression symptoms in women with pelvic floor dysfunction: a case-control study." *Int J Womens Health.* Volume 11:143-148.

44. Ghetti C, Skoczylas LC, Oliphant SS, Nikolajski C, Lowder JL. 2015. "The emotional burden of pelvic organ prolapse in women seeking treatment." *Female Pelvic Med Reconstr Surg.* 21*(6)*:332-338.

45. Brandt C, Janse van Vuuren EC. 2019. "Dysfunction, activity limitations, participation restriction and contextual factors in South African women with pelvic organ prolapse." *South African J Physiother.* 75*(1)*.

46. Mirskaya M, Lindgren E-C, Carlsson I-M. 2019. "Online reported women's experiences of symptomatic pelvic organ prolapse after vaginal birth." *BMC Womens Health.* 19*(1)*:129.

47. Muller N. Pelvic organ prolapse: a patient-centred perspective on what women encounter seeking diagnosis and treatment. Aust New Zeal Cont J. 2010;16*(3)*:70-80.

48. Swenson CW, DePorre JA, Haefner JK, Berger MB, Fenner DE. 2018. "Postpartum depression screening and pelvic floor symptoms among women referred to a specialty postpartum perineal clinic." *Am J Obstet Gynecol.* 218*(3)*:335.e1-335.e6.

49. Webb S, Sherburn M, Ismail KMK. 2014. "Managing perineal trauma after childbirth." *BMJ.* 349*(nov25 27)*:g6829-g6829.

50. Leader-Cramer A, Kenton K, Davé B, Gossett DR, Mueller M, Le-wicky-Gaupp C. 2016. "Factors associated with timing of return to intercourse after obstetric anal sphincter injuries." *J Sex Med.* 13*(10)*:1523-1529.

51. Handelzalts JE, Yaakobi T, Levy S, Peled Y, Wiznitzer A, Krissi H. 2017. "The impact of genital self-image on sexual function in women with pelvic floor disorders." *Eur J Obstet Gynecol Reprod Biol.* 211:164-168.

52. Pizarro-Berdichevsky J, Hitschfeld MJ, Pattillo A, Blumel B, Gonzalez S, Arellano M, Cuevas R, Alvo J, Gorodischer A, Flores-Espinoza C, Goldman HB. 2016. "Association between pelvic floor disorder symptoms and QoL scores with depressive symptoms among pelvic organ prolapse patients." *Aust New Zeal J Obstet Gynaecol.* 56*(4)*:391-397.

53. Wilton G, Moberg DP, Fleming MF. 2009. "The effect of brief alcohol intervention on postpartum depression. *MCN, Am J Matern Nurs.* 34*(5)*:297-302.

54. Meyer I, Richter HE. 2015. "Impact of fecal incontinence and its treatment on quality of life in women." *Women's Heal.* 11*(2)*:225-238.

55. Kegel AH, Powell TO. 1950. "The physiologic treatment of urinary stress incontinence." *J Urol.* 63*(5)*:808-814.

56. Dumoulin C, Cacciari LP, Hay-Smith EJC. 2018. "Pelvic floor muscle training versus no treatment, or inactive control treatments, for urinary incontinence in women." *Cochrane Database Syst Rev.* October 2018.

57. Cammu H, Van Nylen M, Amy JJ. 2000. "A 10-year follow-up after Kegel pelvic floor muscle exercises for genuine stress incontinence." *BJU Int.* 85*(6)*:655-658.

58. Miller JM, Ashton-Miller JA, DeLancey JOL. 1998. "A pelvic muscle precontraction can reduce cough-related urine loss in selected women with mild SUI." *J Am Geriatr Soc.* 46*(7)*:870-874.

59. Elia G, Bergman A. 1993. "Pelvic muscle exercises: When do they work?" *Obstet Gynecol.* 81*(2)*:283-286.

60. Cavkaytar S, Kokanali MK, Topcu HO, Aksakal OS, Doganay M. 2015. "Effect of home-based Kegel exercises on quality of life in women with stress and mixed urinary incontinence." *J Obstet Gynaecol (Lahore).* *35(4)*:407-410.

61. Barney A. 2018. "The mystery of the pelvic floor." *BBC Future.* https://www.bbc.com/future/article/20180717-the-pelvic-floor-is-still-a-mystery-in-anatomy. July 17, 2018.

62. Li C, Gong Y, Wang B. 2016. "The efficacy of pelvic floor muscle training for pelvic organ prolapse: a systematic review and meta-analysis." *Int Urogynecol J.* *27(7)*:981-992.

63. Wallace SL, Miller LD, Mishra K. 2019. "Pelvic floor physical therapy in the treatment of pelvic floor dysfunction in women." *Curr Opin Obstet Gynecol.* *31(6)*:485-493.

64. Saunders K. 2017. "Recent advances in understanding pelvic-floor tissue of women with and without pelvic organ prolapse: Considerations for physical therapists." *Phys Ther.* *97(4)*:455-463.

65. Brookbush B. 2020. "Intrinsic stabilization subsystem integration." https://brookbushinstitute.com/article/intrinsic-stabilization-subsystem/. Accessed June 2020.

66. Kruger J, Budgett D, Goodman J, Bø K. 2019. "Can you train the pelvic floor muscles by contracting other related muscles?" *Neurourol Urodyn.* *38(2)*:677-683.

67. Lee K. 2019. "Investigation of electromyographic activity of pelvic floor muscles in different body positions to prevent urinary incontinence." 25:9357-9363.

68. Stüpp L, Resende APM, Petricelli CD, Nakamura MU, Alexandre SM, Zanetti MRD. 2011. "Pelvic floor muscle and transversus abdominis activation in abdominal hypopressive technique through surface electromyography." *Neurourol Urodyn.* *30(8)*:1518-1521.

69. Navarro Brazález B, Sánchez Sánchez B, Prieto Gómez V, De La Villa Polo P, McLean L, Torres Lacomba M. 2020. "Pelvic floor and abdomi-

nal muscle responses during hypopressive exercises in women with pelvic floor dysfunction." *Neurourol Urodyn.* 39(2):793-803.

70. Juez L, Núñez-Córdoba JM, Couso N, Aubá M, Alcázar JL, Mínguez JÁ. 2019. "Hypopressive technique versus pelvic floor muscle training for postpartum pelvic floor rehabilitation: A prospective cohort study." *Neurourol Urodyn.* 38(7):1924-1931.

71. Resende APM, Bernardes BT, Stüpp L, Oliveira E, Castro RA, Girão MJBC, Sartori MGF. 2019. "Pelvic floor muscle training is better than hypopressive exercises in pelvic organ prolapse treatment: An assessor-blinded randomized controlled trial." *Neurourol Urodyn.* 38(1):171-179.

72. Kissler K, Yount SM, Rendeiro M, Zeidenstein L. 2016. "Primary prevention of urinary incontinence: A case study of prenatal and intrapartum interventions. *J Midwifery Womens Health.* 61(4):507-511.

73. Harvey M-A. 2003. "Pelvic floor exercises during and after pregnancy: A systematic review of their role in preventing pelvic floor dysfunction." *J Obstet Gynaecol Canada.* 25(6):487-498.

74. Liu D, Hu W-L. 2019. "SLK triple therapy improves maternal and fetal status and promotes postpartum pelvic floor function in Chinese primiparous women." *Med Sci Monit.* 25:8913-8919.

75. Varghese C, Wells CI, O'Grady G, Bissett IP. 2020. "Costs and outcomes of sacral nerve stimulation for faecal incontinence in New Zealand: a 10-year observational study." *ANZ J Surg.* 90(4):569-575.

76. Simillis C, Lal N, Qiu S, Kontovounisios C, Rasheed S, Tan E, Tekkis PP. 2018. "Sacral nerve stimulation versus percutaneous tibial nerve stimulation for faecal incontinence: a systematic review and meta-analysis." *Int J Colorectal Dis.* 33(5):645-648.

77. Noblett KL, Cadish LA. 2014. "Sacral nerve stimulation for the treatment of refractory voiding and bowel dysfunction." *Am J Obstet Gynecol.* 210(2):99-106.

78. Palus S. 2019. "Are you Kegel-ing correctly?" *Slate.* September 2019. https://slate.com/human-interest/2019/09/kegel-bluetooth-devices-stop-incontinence-better-sex.html.

79. Barbalat Y, Tunuguntla HSGR. 2012. "Surgery for pelvic organ prolapse: A historical perspective." *Curr Urol Rep.* 13*(3)*:256-261.

80. Hasan I, Zulkifle M, Ansari AH, Sherwani AMK, Shakir M. 2011. "History of ancient Egyptian obstetrics & gynecology: A review." *J Microbiol Biotech Res.* 1*(1)*:35-39.

81. Downing KT. 2012. "Uterine prolapse: From antiquity to today." *Obstet Gynecol Int.* 2012:1-9.

82. Carvalho C, da Silva Serrão PRM, Beleza ACS, Driusso P. 2020. "Pelvic floor dysfunctions in female cheerleaders: a cross-sectional study." *Int Urogynecol J.* 31*(5)*:999-1006.

83. Larsen WI, Yavorek T. 2007. "Pelvic prolapse and urinary incontinence in nulliparous college women in relation to paratrooper training." *Int Urogynecol J.* 18*(7)*:769-771.

84. Yang J, Cheng JW, Wagner H, Lohman E, Yang SH, Krishingner GA, Trofimova A, Alsyouf M, Staack A. 2019. "The effect of high impact crossfit exercises on stress urinary incontinence in physically active women." *Neurourol Urodyn.* 38*(2)*:749-756.

85. Brennand E, Ruiz-Mirazo E, Tang S, Kim-Fine S. 2018. "Urinary leakage during exercise: problematic activities, adaptive behaviors, and interest in treatment for physically active Canadian women." *Int Urogynecol J.* 29*(4)*:497-503.

86. Kruger JA, Dietz HP, Murphy BA. 2007. "Pelvic floor function in elite nulliparous athletes." *Ultrasound Obstet Gynecol.* 30*(1)*:81-85.

87. Bø K, Nygaard IE. 2020. "Is physical activity good or bad for the female pelvic floor? A narrative review." *Sport Med.* 50*(3)*:471-484.

88. Ali-Ross N, Smith A, Hosker G. 2009. "The effect of physical activity on pelvic organ prolapse." *BJOG An Int J Obstet Gynaecol.* 116*(6)*:824-828.

89. FDA. 2019. "Surgical mesh for transvaginal repair of pelvic organ prolapse in the anterior vaginal compartment." *FDA Executive Summary.* https://www.fda.gov/media/122854/download.

90. Von Bargen EC, Hudson PL, Berkowitz LR. 2019. "Vaginal hysterectomy, uterosacral ligament suspension, anterior repair, and perineorrhaphy." *J Med Insight. (267).*

91. Ortega M V., Von Bargen EC, Bordeianou LG. 2019. "Laparoscopic suture rectopexy with culdoplasty, vaginal wall repair, and perineorrhaphy for rectal prolapse." *J Med Insight. (272).*

92. Arenholt LTS, Pedersen BG, Glavind K, Glavind-Kristensen M, DeLancey JOL. 2017. "Paravaginal defect: anatomy, clinical findings, and imaging." *Int Urogynecol J. 28(5)*:661-673.

93. Zuchelo LTS, Bezerra IMP, Da Silva ATM, Gomes JM,1,4 Soares Jr JM, Baracat EC, de Abreu LC, Sorpresol ICE. 2018. "Questionnaires to evaluate pelvic floor dysfunction in the postpartum period: a systematic review." *Int J Womens Health.* Volume 10:409-424.

94. Zhu YC, Deng SH, Jiang Q, Zhang Y. 2018. "Correlation between delivery mode and pelvic organ prolapse evaluated by four-dimensional pelvic floor ultrasonography." *Med Sci Monit.* 24:7891-7897.

95. Liu Y-J, Wu W-Y, Hsiao S-M, Ting SW-H, Hsu H-P, Huang C-M. 2018. "Efficacy of pelvic floor training with surface electromyography feedback for female stress urinary incontinence." *Int J Nurs Pract. 24(6)*:e12698.

96. Moretti E, de Moura Filho AG, de Almeida JC, Araujo CM, Lemos A. 2017. "Electromyographic assessment of women's pelvic floor: What is the best place for a superficial sensor?" *Neurourol Urodyn. 36(7)*:1917-1923.

97. Bohorquez J, McKinney J, Keyser L, Sutherland R, Pulliam SJ. 2020. "Development of a wireless accelerometer-based Intravaginal device to detect pelvic floor motion for evaluation of pelvic floor dysfunction." *Biomed Microdevices. 22(2)*:26.

98. Grahame R. 1999. "Joint hypermobility and genetic collagen disorders: Are they related?" *Arch Dis Child.* 80*(2)*:188-191.

99. Hafizi L, Mirfeizi Z, Razmjoo N, Keshvari M, Jabbari A, Ashraf H, Yousefi F. 2013. "The association between women's pelvic organ prolapse and joint hypermobility." *J Pak Med Assoc.* 63*(9)*:1152-1156.

100. Veit-Rubin N, Cartwright R, Singh AU, Digesu GA, Fernando R, Khullar V. 2016. "Association between joint hypermobility and pelvic organ prolapse in women: a systematic review and meta-analysis." *Int Urogynecol J.* 27*(10)*:1469-1478.

101. Li XJ, Pan HT, Chen JJ, Fu YB, Fang M, He GH, Zhang T, Ding HG, Yu B, Cheng Y, Tan YJ, Zhao FL, Morse AN, Huang HF. 2019. "Proteomics of uterosacral ligament connective tissue from women with and without pelvic organ prolapse." *Proteomics - Clin Appl.* 13*(4)*:1-8.

102. Halverson AL. 2005. "Nonoperative management of fecal incontinence." *Clin Colon Rectal Surg.* 18*(01)*:17-21.

ILLUSTRATION CREDITS

Cover design by MiblArt.

Cover photos by GaryAlvis/iStock and BLACKDAY/Shuttershock.

Author photo by Michael Poole.

Page 13) Adapted from an illustration by Alila Medical Media/Shutterstock.

Page 122) Illustration by Paul Riss and Wolfgang Umek. From "Anatomical Landmarks in the Small Pelvis," presented at the 2010 Annual Meeting of the International Continence Society and International Urogynecological Association. Modified by author.

Page 123) By Mikael Häggström, used with permission.

Page 126) Illustration from page 560 of "The Principles and practice of gynecology : for students and practitioners" (1904) by Emilius Clark Dudley. Via Internet Archive Book Images on Flickr. Modified by author.

Page 127) Illustration from page 109 of "The diseases of women : a handbook for students and practitioners" (1897) by Sir John Bland-Sutton and Arthur Edward Giles. Via Internet Archive Book Images on Flickr.

Page 128) Illustration from page 109 of "The diseases of women : a handbook for students and practitioners" (1897) by Sir John Bland-Sutton and Arthur Edward Giles. Via Internet Archive Book Images on Flickr.

Page 149) Photo by author.

APPENDIX A

ANATOMY
OF THE
PELVIC FLOOR

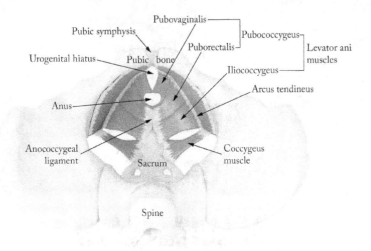

THE PELVIC DIAPHRAGM

This image shows uninjured pelvic floor muscles in the female pelvis. We are looking into the pelvis from inside the body. The muscles of the pelvic floor form a bowl to support your organs. Notice that there is no muscular support for the vaginal or urethral opening. This hole, needed for voiding urine, sexual intercourse, and giving birth, is called the urogenital hiatus.

There are three muscle bands of the levator ani muscles: pubovaginalis, puborectalis, and iliococcygeus. The pubovaginalis muscle forms an arch around the urogenital hiatus and contracts to close the hiatus. The puborectalis forms an arched sling around the rectum and contracts to hold the rectum at an angle and prevent the passage of stool. All three bands of levator ani muscles attach to the arcus tendineus ligament.

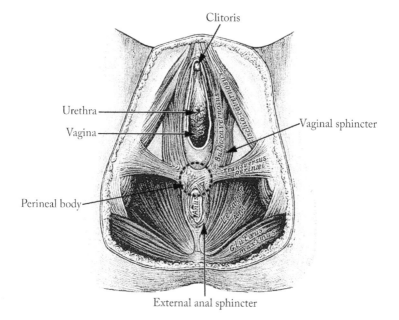

Clitoris

Urethra

Vagina

Vaginal sphincter

Perineal body

External anal sphincter

THE PERINEAL BODY

Here we are looking at the female pelvis from outside the body. This image shows the superficial pelvic muscles, located between the pelvic floor and the skin. The perineal body, indicated with the dotted circle, is the central tendinous anchor point for the superficial muscles, and an integration point between the superficial muscles and the deeper levator ani muscles. The vaginal sphincter (AKA the bulbospongiosus, and previously as the bulbocavernosus) functions to constrict the vaginal opening and to compress the vestibular bulb *(female erectile tissue)*. The transverse perineal muscle stabilizes the perineal body. The external anal sphincter is a ring of skeletal muscle around the anus that is under voluntary control. The sphincter contracts to hold the anus shut and block the passage of stool.

PELVIC ORGAN PROLAPSE (POP)

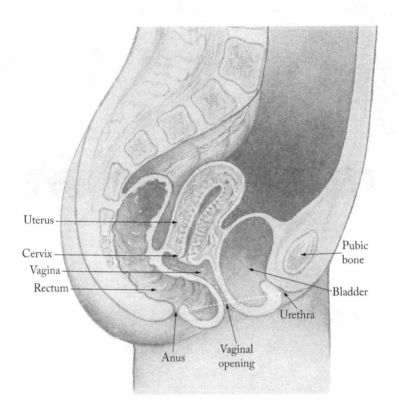

Uterus

Cervix

Vagina

Rectum

Pubic bone

Bladder

Urethra

Anus

Vaginal opening

ANTERIOR AND POSTERIOR PROLAPSE, INTERNAL VIEW

This image shows the pelvis of a woman with prolapse of the bladder and rectum. As you can see, both bladder and rectum are invading the vaginal space. Everything below the dotted line is protruding outside of the vaginal opening. Pooling of urine and feces would occur in the bulges extending below the dotted line, where the rectum is below the anus and the bladder is below the urethra. The uterus is slightly lower than normal, being pulled down by its attachment to the bladder and rectum. By POP-Q staging criteria, this woman has stage II anterior and posterior prolapse, as well as stage I uterine prolapse.

KEGELS ARE NOT GOING TO FIX THIS | 127

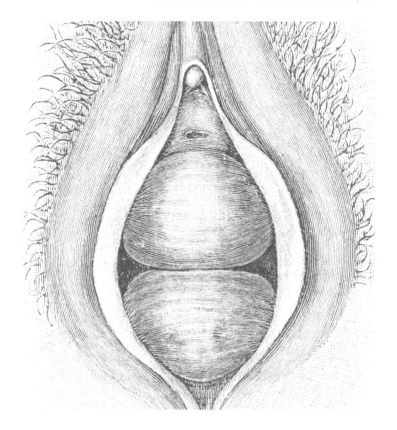

ANTERIOR AND POSTERIOR PROLAPSE, EXTERNAL VIEW

Here is what a woman presenting with stage II anterior and posterior prolapse as in Fig. 3 might look like from the outside.

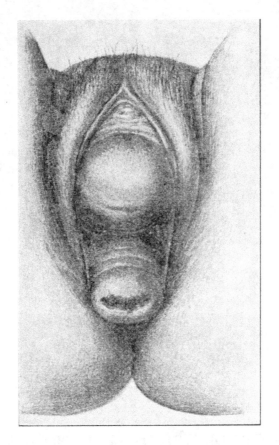

ANTERIOR AND UTERINE PROLAPSE, EXTERNAL VIEW

Here is what a woman presenting with stage III anterior and uterine prolapse might look like from the outside. The bladder is bulging into the anterior vaginal wall and the uterus has descended. Both the bulge and the cervix are visible, extending outside of the vaginal opening.

TIPS AND TRICKS FOR PELVIC FLOOR DISORDER RELIEF

HYPOALLERGENIC VULVAR CARE

These instructions will help you to reduce exposure of your sensitive vulvar and perineal tissues to common allergens. By strictly following these precautions, you will likely see at least some improvement in the burning, itching and/or pain you experience in these areas. A barrier cream, such as zinc oxide, may also be helpful in the prevention of skin irritation.

It is very important not to scratch these sensitive tissues. Using an over the counter hydrocortisone cream during flareups can be helpful. You can find these next to the yeast infection creams. During a flareup, apply the cream to external genitals 2 or 3 times a day for several days. Then reduce to once a day for several days. Then stop. Ice packs are also effective at reducing itching and pain. If itching is severe, try an antihistamine.

- Use a fragrance free, hypoallergic body soap *(e.g. Basis, Aveeno, Dove for sensitive skin)*

- Use a laundry detergent that is free of dyes and perfumes to launder your clothes. Do not use fabric softeners or anti-cling agents.

- Avoid exposing vulvar tissues to shampoo and conditioner. Use the handheld shower nozzle and bend forward while rinsing your hair or wear swimsuit bottoms in the shower.

- If you take a bath, keep the water free of irritants. Do not shampoo and condition your hair while in the tub and do not use bubbles or bath bombs.

- Wear cotton underwear or at least underwear with a 100% cotton crotch panel except when planning to work up a sweat. Then wear a wicking synthetic fabric like nylon and switch back to fresh cotton pair as soon as possible after exercise.

- Use unscented incontinence or sanitary pads, ideally that have at least a top layer of cotton.

- Use unscented toilet paper that does not leave lint behind *(e.g. Angel Soft)*. Lint is the enemy. Always pat dry instead of rubbing.

- Better yet, use hypoallergenic baby wipes *(e.g. Water Wipes)* or purchase a handheld/travel bidet and use a squirt of water to clean. Pat dry with a towel.

- Take a calcium supplement *(1500 milligrams per day)*.

- Use lubrication during intercourse *(e.g. Uber Lube, Astro-glide, or Slippery Stuff)*.

- Do not shave off pubic hair.

GETTING URINE OUT

Damage to the pelvic floor can make it more difficult to void your bladder completely. If you notice that urine continues to dribble out after you have finished actively urinating, you may be having this problem.

The following will help you to get more of your urine out. Sit on the toilet seat *(don't hover over it)* with your feet flat on the ground. As you are urinating, try leaning forward. If you are still dribbling, you can even try going into a forward fold and lifting your bottom slightly off the seat, such that your bottom is higher than your urethra. Think of your bladder as a pitcher full of water, and you need to pour all the water out.

You can also try waiting for ten seconds or more after you are done urinating. Stand up and sit back down again. Lean forward and back. Then try again. Sometimes these movements get the urine closer to the "spout" so that it is easier to get out.

Lastly, you can try giving your bladder a manual assist. Tilt forward slightly, reach your hand behind you, and gently push up on your perineum and vagina with your palm. This is especially helpful for those with prolapse of the bladder. Pushing up on the bulge can help urine reach the exit.

GETTING FECES OUT

You may be constipated. Be sure to take a daily fiber supplement with the active ingredient psyllium fiber. Drink plenty of water and chew your food adequately. Walking can help prepare the body for bowel movements.

Sit on the toilet, don't hover. Place your feet on a stool to create a better angle for the poop to get out. If no stool is available, you can create a similar angle by lifting your heels up so that your knees are raised. Try rocking the top half of your body back and forth and side to side.

Do not hold your breath or strain while pooping. Try taking slow deep breaths that expand your diaphragm and your stomach, then give a gentle push on the exhale. You can also try blowing into a fisted hand during exhale.

If you have prolapse, your feces may be getting stuck in your prolapsed rectum. Before you start to push, make a thumbs up sign, reach your hand down between your legs, and stick your thumb into your vagina with the pad of your thumb facing toward the back. Push gently on the posterior *(back)* wall to brace the hernia while you poop. If you don't like using your thumb, you can purchase femmeze, a product designed to serve this function.

KEEPING URINE AND FECES IN

The sensation of urgency can make leakage more likely. Try avoiding or minimizing foods and beverages that increase urgency. Caffeine and alcohol are irritants that increase urgency and cause loose stool. For many there is a threshold effect and keeping your daily intake within limits is sufficient to reduce urgency. For caffeine, an upper limit of 250 milligrams a day is a useful guideline. For alcohol, drinking in moderation *(1-2 servings)* and taking at least a few days off from drinking alcohol a week can improve urgency. For others caffeine and alcohol must be eliminated from the diet entirely to see an improvement.

Additional common irritants include citrus, carbonated beverages, artificial sweeteners, milk products, and spicy food. Identifying your irritants and eliminating them from your diet or reducing your intake may improve problems with urgency.

If you are feeling an urgent need to go, try contracting your pelvic floor muscles and/or external sphincter several times as fast as you can. For some women, this trick stops urgency long enough that they can make it to the restroom.

Weight loss can reduce leakage caused by urinary and fecal incontinence.

Diarrhea is more likely to leak out. Taking a daily fiber supplement with the active ingredient psyllium fiber along with each meal can increase the bulk of your stool.

Bladder retraining may be useful for women who urinate frequently and who need to get up to urinate more than once a night *(a problem called nocturia)*. You can learn more about this from the resources listed at the end of this section.

STRATEGIES FOR WOMEN WITH FECAL INCONTINENCE

From what I have read, you are probably already hyperaware of your bowel habits. If you haven't already, try keeping a journal of what you eat and when you eat it as well as when you have bowel movements. The goal of the journal is to work toward regularity, so that you have bowel movements at rougly the same time each day and can predict when you will need a restroom. This is called bowel training.

You can reduce the risk of leakage by giving yourself an enema as needed. In "Nonoperative Management of Fecal Incontinence," Dr. Halverson wrote, "Self-administering an enema before participating in active physical exercise or sexual relations may give an individual more confidence in these potentially stressful situations. For those individuals who experience post-defecation leakage, taking a tap water enema just after a bowel movement may help to cleanse the rectal vault and decrease any seepage that may occur following a bowel movement."[102]

REST

Sitting or standing for a long time can increase discomfort. Be sure to alternate between positions if possible. I found that switching between sitting and standing on a wobble board helps me a lot during a long day at my computer.

Find a restful position that provides relief from the pressure of pelvic floor disorders. One physical therapist recommended option is to lie down and place a few pillows under your butt, so that your pelvis is elevated. Get comfortable with a book or your phone and sit like this for twenty minutes at least once a day. I like to sit like this and put my feet up the wall. I found that this trick provides a lot of relief.

Other positions I have found soothing are child's pose, downward facing dog, and doggy style position *(minus the partner)*. That is, butt in the air, knees, elbows, forearms, and forehead on the floor.

ONLINE RESOURCES

Voices for PFD is the best public facing website on pelvic floor disorders. It was created by the American Urogynecologic Society. All advice is evidence-based and trustworthy.

- voicesforpfd.org

The National Vulvodynia Association has a website on vulvodynia, with information for patients and women's health professionals.

- nva.org

The Vulval Pain Society has a public facing website for those who suffer from vulvar pain, created by a doctor and nurse.

- vulvalpainsociety.org

- UpToDate has excellent summary articles on pelvic floor disorders, regularly updated to include the latest research. The following links go to free, public facing summaries.

- Fecal incontinence: uptodate.com/contents/fecal-incontinence-beyond-the-basics

- Urinary incontinence: uptodate.com/contents/urinary-incontinence-in-women-beyond-the-basics

- Pelvic floor muscle exercises: uptodate.com/contents/pelvic-floor-muscle-exercises-beyond-the-basics

- Sexual problems: uptodate.com/contents/sexual-problems-in-women-beyond-the-basics

PELVIC HEALTH AND QUALITY OF LIFE QUESTIONNAIRES

The following questionnaires are commonly used to assess the severity of any pelvic floor disorder symptoms you may have and how they are affecting your quality of life. They are included here as a tool for self-assessment, and to prepare you for meeting with your doctor. These forms give you the language to use when you discuss your symptoms. If your symptoms are having a negative impact on your quality of life, be sure to say so. If your regular doctor does not seem to know much about pelvic floor disorders, ask to be referred to a urogynecologist.

PELVIC HEALTH
PELVIC FLOOR DISABILITY INDEX (PFDI-20)

Instructions: Please answer all of the questions in the following survey. These questions will ask you if you have certain bowel, bladder, or pelvic symptoms and, if you do, how much they bother you on a scale from 1 to 4. Answer these by circling the appropriate number. While answering these questions, please consider your symptoms over the last 3 months.

Pelvic Organ prolapse Distress Inventory 6 (POPDI-6)

Do You...	NO	YES
1. Usually experience pressure in the lower abdomen?	0	1 2 3 4
2. Usually experience heaviness or dullness in the pelvic area?	0	1 2 3 4
3. Usually have a bulge or something falling out that you can see or feel in your vaginal area?	0	1 2 3 4
4. Ever have to push on the vagina or around the rectum to have or complete a bowel movement?	0	1 2 3 4
5. Usually experience a feeling of incomplete bladder emptying?	0	1 2 3 4
6. Ever have to push up on a bulge in the vaginal area with your fingers to start or complete urination?	0	1 2 3 4

Colorectal-Anal distress Inventory 8 (CRAD-8)

Do You...	NO	YES
7. Feel you need to strain too hard to have a bowel movement?	0	1 2 3 4
8. Feel you have not completely emptied your bowels at the end of a bowel movement?	0	1 2 3 4
9. Usually lose stool beyond your control if your stool is well formed?	0	1 2 3 4
10. Usually lose stool beyond your control if your stool is loose?	0	1 2 3 4
11. Usually lose gas from the rectum beyond your control?	0	1 2 3 4
12. Usually have pain when you pass your stool?	0	1 2 3 4
13. Experience a strong sense of urgency and have to rush to the bathroom to have a bowel movement?	0	1 2 3 4
14. Does part of your bowel ever pass through the rectum and bulge outside during or after a bowel movement?	0	1 2 3 4

Urinary distress Inventory 6 (UDI-6)

Do You...	NO	YES
15. Usually experience frequent urination?	0	1 2 3 4
16. Usually experience urine leakage associated with a feeling of urgency, that is, a strong sensation of needing to go to the bathroom?	0	1 2 3 4
17. Usually experience urine leakage related to coughing, sneezing or laughing?	0	1 2 3 4
18. Usually experience small amounts of urine leakage (that is, drops)?	0	1 2 3 4
19. Usually experience difficulty emptying your bladder?	0	1 2 3 4
20. Usually experience pain or discomfort in the lower abdomen or genital region?	0	1 2 3 4

SEXUAL HEALTH
SEXUAL FUNCTION FOR WOMEN WITH PELVIC ORGAN PROLAPSE, URINARY INCONTINENCE, AND/OR FECAL INCONTINENCE (PISQ-IR)

By the International Urogynecological Association

Source: https://www.iuga.org/resources/pisq-ir

Q1   Which of the following best describes you:

Not sexually active at all   1 ☐ ➔   Go to item Q2 (Section 1)

Sexually active <u>with or without</u> a partner   2 ☐ ➔   Skip to item Q7 (Section 2)

Section 1: For those who are not Sexually Active

☞ If you engage in sexual activity please check this box ☐ and skip to Page 3

Q2 The following are a list of reasons why you might not be <u>sexually active</u>, for each one please indicate how strongly you agree or disagree with it as a <u>reason that you are not sexually active.</u>

	STRONGLY AGREE	SOMEWHAT AGREE	SOMEWHAT DISAGREE	STRONGLY DISAGREE
a No partner	☐¹	☐²	☐³	☐⁴
b No Interest	☐¹	☐²	☐³	☐⁴
c Due to bladder or bowel problems (urinary or fecal incontinence) or due to prolapse (a feeling of or a bulge in the vaginal area)	☐¹	☐²	☐³	☐⁴
d Because of my other health problems	☐¹	☐²	☐³	☐⁴
e Pain	☐¹	☐²	☐³	☐⁴

Q3 How much does the <u>fear</u> of leaking urine and/or stool and/or a bulging in the vagina (either the bladder, rectum or uterus falling out) cause you to <u>avoid or restrict</u> your sexual activity?

1 ☐ Not at All
2 ☐ A Little
3 ☐ Some
4 ☐ A Lot

Q4 For each of the following, <u>please circle the number between 1 and 5</u> that best represents how you feel about your sex life.

		RATING					
a.	Satisfied	1	2	3	4	5	Dissatisfied
b.	Adequate	1	2	3	4	5	Inadequate

Q5 How strongly do you agree or disagree with each of the following statements:

	STRONGLY AGREE	SOMEWHAT AGREE	SOMEWHAT DISAGREE	STRONGLY DISAGREE
a. I feel frustrated by my sex life	☐¹	☐²	☐³	☐⁴
b. I feel sexually inferior because of my incontinence and/or prolapse	☐¹	☐²	☐³	☐⁴
c. I feel angry because of the impact that incontinence and/or prolapse has on my sex life	☐¹	☐²	☐³	☐⁴

Q6 Overall, how bothersome is it to you that you are not sexually active?

1 ☐ Not at All
2 ☐ A Little
3 ☐ Some
4 ☐ A Lot

End of Items for Not Sexually Active

Section 2: For Those Who are Sexually Active

The remaining items in the survey are about a topic that one is not often asked to report on in a survey please answer as honestly and clearly as you possibly can.

Q7   How often do you feel sexually aroused (physically excited or turned on) during sexual activity?

    1 ☐ Never
    2 ☐ Rarely
    3 ☐ Sometimes
    4 ☐ Usually
    5 ☐ Always

Q8   When you are involved in sexual activity, how often do you feel each of the following:

	NEVER	RARELY	SOMETIMES	USUALLY	ALMOST ALWAYS
a. Fulfilled	☐¹	☐²	☐³	☐⁴	☐⁵
b. Shame	☐¹	☐²	☐³	☐⁴	☐⁵
c. Fear	☐¹	☐²	☐³	☐⁴	☐⁵

Q9   How often do you leak urine and/or stool with any type of sexual activity?

    1 ☐ Never
    2 ☐ Rarely
    3 ☐ Sometimes
    4 ☐ Usually
    5 ☐ Always

Q10   Compared to orgasms you have had in the past, how intense are your orgasms now?

    1 ☐ Much less intense
    2 ☐ Less intense
    3 ☐ Same intensity
    4 ☐ More intense
    5 ☐ Much more intense

Q11   How often do you feel pain during sexual intercourse? (If you don't have intercourse check this box ☐ and skip to the next item.)

    1 ☐ Never
    2 ☐ Rarely
    3 ☐ Sometimes
    4 ☐ Usually
    5 ☐ Always

Q12   Do you have a sexual partner?

    1 ☐ Yes ➜ Go to Q13
    2 ☐ No ➜ Skip to Q15

Q13   How often does your partner have a problem (lack of arousal, desire, erection ,etc.) that limits your sexual activity?

    1 ☐ All of the time
    2 ☐ Most of the time
    3 ☐ Some of the time
    4 ☐ Hardly ever/Rarely

Q14   In general, would you say that your partner has a positive or negative impact on each of the following:

	VERY POSITIVE	SOMEWHAT POSITIVE	SOMEWHAT NEGATIVE	VERY NEGATIVE
a. Your sexual desire	☐¹	☐²	☐³	☐⁴
b. The frequency of your sexual activity	☐¹	☐²	☐³	☐⁴

Q15 When you are involved in sexual activity, how often do you feel that you want more?

1 ☐ Never
2 ☐ Rarely
3 ☐ Sometimes
4 ☐ Usually
5 ☐ Always

Q16 How frequently do you have sexual desire, this may include wanting to have sex, having sexual thoughts or fantasies, etc.?

1 ☐ Daily
2 ☐ Weekly
3 ☐ Monthly
4 ☐ Less often than once a Month
5 ☐ Never

Q17 How would you rate your level (degree) of sexual desire or interest?

1 ☐ Very high
2 ☐ High
3 ☐ Moderate
4 ☐ Low
5 ☐ Very low or none at all

Q18 How much does the fear of leaking urine, stool and/or a bulging in the vagina(prolapse) cause you to avoid sexual activity?

1 ☐ Not at All
2 ☐ A Little
3 ☐ Some
4 ☐ A Lot

Q19 For each of the following, please circle the number between 1 and 5 that best represents how you feel about your sex life.

				RATING			
a	Satisfied	1	2	3	4	5	Dissatisfied
b	Adequate	1	2	3	4	5	Inadequate
c	Confident	1	2	3	4	5	Not Confident

Q20 How strongly do you agree or disagree with each of the following statements.

	STRONGLY AGREE	SOMEWHAT AGREE	SOMEWHAT DISAGREE	STRONGLY DISAGREE
a. I feel frustrated by my sex life	☐[1]	☐[2]	☐[3]	☐[4]
b. I feel sexually inferior because of my incontinence and/or prolapse	☐[1]	☐[2]	☐[3]	☐[4]
c. I feel embarrassed about my sex life	☐[1]	☐[2]	☐[3]	☐[4]
d. I feel angry because of the impact that incontinence and/or prolapse has on my sex life	☐[1]	☐[2]	☐[3]	☐[4]

QUALITY OF LIFE
PELVIC FLOOR IMPACT QUESTIONNAIRE
SHORT FORM 7 (PFIQ-7)

Instructions: Some women find that bladder, bowel, or vaginal symptoms affect their activities, relationships, and feelings. For each question, check the response that best describes how much your activities, relationships, or feelings have been affected by your bladder, bowel and vaginal / pelvic symptoms or conditions over the last 3 months. Please be sure to mark an answer in all 3 columns for each question.

How do symptoms or conditions in the following usually affect your	Bladder or Urine	Bowel or Rectum	Vagina or Pelvis
1. Ability to do household chores (cooking, laundry housecleaning)?	☐ Not at all ☐ Somewhat ☐ Moderately ☐ Quite a bit	☐ Not at all ☐ Somewhat ☐ Moderately ☐ Quite a bit	☐ Not at all ☐ Somewhat ☐ Moderately ☐ Quite a bit
2. Ability to do physical activities such as walking, swimming, or other exercise?	☐ Not at all ☐ Somewhat ☐ Moderately ☐ Quite a bit	☐ Not at all ☐ Somewhat ☐ Moderately ☐ Quite a bit	☐ Not at all ☐ Somewhat ☐ Moderately ☐ Quite a bit
3. Entertainment activities such as going to a movie or concert?	☐ Not at all ☐ Somewhat ☐ Moderately ☐ Quite a bit	☐ Not at all ☐ Somewhat ☐ Moderately ☐ Quite a bit	☐ Not at all ☐ Somewhat ☐ Moderately ☐ Quite a bit
4. Ability to travel by car or bus for a distance greater than 30 minutes away from home?	☐ Not at all ☐ Somewhat ☐ Moderately ☐ Quite a bit	☐ Not at all ☐ Somewhat ☐ Moderately ☐ Quite a bit	☐ Not at all ☐ Somewhat ☐ Moderately ☐ Quite a bit
5. Participating in social activities outside your home?	☐ Not at all ☐ Somewhat ☐ Moderately ☐ Quite a bit	☐ Not at all ☐ Somewhat ☐ Moderately ☐ Quite a bit	☐ Not at all ☐ Somewhat ☐ Moderately ☐ Quite a bit
6. Emotional health (nervousness, depression, etc.)?	☐ Not at all ☐ Somewhat ☐ Moderately ☐ Quite a bit	☐ Not at all ☐ Somewhat ☐ Moderately ☐ Quite a bit	☐ Not at all ☐ Somewhat ☐ Moderately ☐ Quite a bit
7. Feeling frustrated?	☐ Not at all ☐ Somewhat ☐ Moderately ☐ Quite a bit	☐ Not at all ☐ Somewhat ☐ Moderately ☐ Quite a bit	☐ Not at all ☐ Somewhat ☐ Moderately ☐ Quite a bit

MENTAL HEALTH
PATIENT HEALTH QUESTIONNAIRE (PHQ-9)

Over the last *2 weeks,* how often have you been bothered by any of the following problems?
(use "✓" to indicate your answer)

	Not at all	Several days	More than half the days	Nearly every day
1. Little interest or pleasure in doing things	0	1	2	3
2. Feeling down, depressed, or hopeless	0	1	2	3
3. Trouble falling or staying asleep, or sleeping too much	0	1	2	3
4. Feeling tired or having little energy	0	1	2	3
5. Poor appetite or overeating	0	1	2	3
6. Feeling bad about yourself - or that you are a failure or have let yourself or your family down	0	1	2	3
7. Trouble concentrating on things, such as reading the newspaper or watching television	0	1	2	3
8. Moving or speaking so slowly that other people could have noticed. Or the opposite - being so fidgety or restless that you have been moving around a lot more than usual	0	1	2	3
9. Thoughts that you would be better off dead, or of hurting yourself	0	1	2	3

add columns ___ + ___ + ___

(Healthcare professional: For interpretation of TOTAL, please refer to accompanying scoring card). TOTAL: _____

10. If you checked off *any problems,* how *difficult* have these problems made it for you to do your work, take care of things at home, or get along with other people?

Not difficult at all _____
Somewhat difficult _____
Very difficult _____
Extremely difficult _____

THANK YOU FOR READING

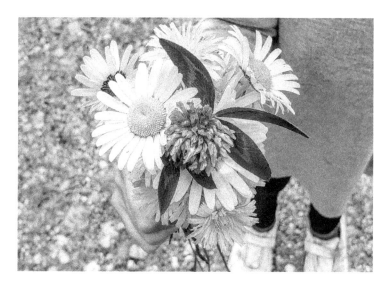

I hope you have found this book to be a useful resource. If you have any questions or comments, please don't hesitate to reach out. You can find my contact information and links to social media accounts on my website.

georgeannsack.com

CPSIA information can be obtained
at www.ICGtesting.com
Printed in the USA
BVHW062301111022
649159BV00018B/1371

9 781735 090405